THE THRIVE DIET

THE THRIVE DIET

the whole food way to lose weight, reduce stress, and stay healthy for life

BRENDAN BRAZIER

Da Capo
LIFE LONG
A Member of the Perseus Books Goup

Originally published in 2007 by the Penguin Group (Canada). This edition published by arrangement with Penguin Canada.

Cataloging-in-Publication data for this book is available from the Library of Congress.

First Da Capo Press edition 2007
ISBN-10: 1-60094-060-9
ISBN-13: 978-1-60094-060-6

Published by Da Capo Press
A Member of the Perseus Books Group
www.dacapopress.com

10 9 8 7 6 5 4 3 2 1

To Lynn, Seymour, and Stanley

contents

Introduction *1*

1 Reduce Stress to Increase Vitality 9

My Introduction to Stress 12

The Toll of Stress 15

Types of Stress 20

2 Understanding the Thrive Diet 33

High Net-Gain Nutrition Is the Key 34

Raw and Low-Temperature Cooked Foods 44

Alkaline-Forming Foods to pH Balance the Body 47

One-Step Nutrition 57

Nutrient-Dense Whole Foods Will Keep You Satisfied 60

Whole Foods for Complete Nourishment 62

Determining Common Food Sensitivities 64

Eliminating Biological Debt 70

Hydration 78

Lifestyle Tips to Complement the Thrive Diet 80

Applying the Thrive Diet 85

Recalibration: Ease into It 88

Getting Started on the Thrive Diet 89

3 The Thrive Diet for a Healthy Environment 92

The Energy Requirements of Food Production 92

Protein Production: A Significant Environmental Strain 95

Soil Quality 96

Why the Thrive Diet Is Less Demanding on the Environment 97

What Can We Do? 98

4 Exercise for Lifelong Health 100

Exercise: Getting Started 102

Proper Nutrition Boosts Exercise's Positive Effects 106

Nutrition Before Exercise 108

Nutrition During Exercise 114

Nutrition Immediately After Exercise 118

Alkalizing Foods and Exercise 121

Exercise-Specific Recipes 122

5 Staple Foods for the Thrive Diet 130

Vegetables 130

Legumes 133

Seeds 134

Pseudograins 139

Fruit 142

Oils 143

Nuts 145

Grains 147

Next-Level Foods 149

Additives 158

6 Meal Plans for the Thrive Diet 161

Shopping List 161

Appliances Needed 164

Traveling and the Thrive Diet 164

The Meal Plan 167

The Thrive Diet 12-Week Meal Plan 169

7 Recipes for the Thrive Diet 200

My Recipe Philosophy 200

Herbs 201

Soaking and Sprouting 202

Variations 205

Recipes 209

Variations 209
Thrive Diet Basics 209
Pancakes 211
Cereals 215
Smoothies 217
Energy Bars 226
Burgers 232
Pizzas 234
Vegetables 240
Soups 244
Salads 246
Salad Dressings 251
Crackers 257
Sauces, Dips, and Spreads 261
Drinks 267
Desserts 269

Appendix 273

Vitamins and Minerals 273

Carbohydrate, Fat, and Protein 281

Glossary 285

Resources 290

References 297

Recipe Index 301

Subject Index 303

introduction

The Thrive Diet grew out of necessity. At the age of 15, I decided that I wanted to become a professional athlete. My goal was to ultimately be a professional Ironman triathlete. Consisting of a 2.4-mile swim, 112-mile cycle, and a 26.2-mile run (a marathon), Ironman triathlon racing is not the easiest way to make a living. But it appealed to me. I enjoyed outdoor exercise, hard work, and a challenge, so why not make a career out of it?

As you can imagine, I needed to dedicate a huge amount of time and effort to training for this event. As I got more serious about training and pursuing my goal, I searched for ways to improve my performance. Not wanting to reinvent the wheel, I looked at how other athletes were training.

What immediately stood out to me was how little their training programs varied. From the top pros in the sport right down to the average performers, the variations in their workout routines were only slight. Taking training out of the equation, then, what then allowed some athletes to improve at an exceptional rate, while others became stagnant or made only modest gains? What separated the top athletes from the average? As I found, there are only two prime components that make up an athlete's routine: training and recovery. Often referred to as stress and rest, both elements are of equal importance, yet usually only one gets attention—the training.

While training programs are meticulously plotted and each workout is planned in detail, little thought is given to recovery. We know that recovery occurs when the body is at rest, but, as I learned, there are varying states of rest that are not well understood. Maximizing the quality of rest is key. Removing other forms of stress from the body during times of rest will speed the rate of recovery. In doing so, the athlete will be better physiologically prepared for the next workout and therefore will benefit from it more. It was the recovery that needed to be my prime focus, not the training.

After reading many articles and speaking with a wide variety of top professional athletes in both strength and endurance, I found that the major variant among athletes was diet. They ranged from very poor to pretty good. So did their performance: The better the diet, the better the recovery rate. But what constituted a good diet? What were the best foods to eat for recovery and which ones should be avoided? Which foods helped the body function in a reduced state of stress so that it could recover faster?

My focus, which had begun on training, now shifted to recovery and, more specifically, diet. I tried different diets, not restrictive ones, as is a common theme of many diets, but supposedly performance-enhancing ones. I tried high-carbohydrate, grain-based, low-fat, low-protein diets, and low-carbohydrate, high-fat, high-protein diets, and several others that fell in between. Although learning the basic principles of the various diets was helpful, I couldn't find any one diet that really gave me the edge I was looking for.

Then I tried a diet that was considered at the time to be a novelty. It was the earlier 1990s and diets that did not consist of meat and dairy products, regardless of their other parameters, were usually dismissed immediately, especially by athletes. But I tried this completely plant-based diet. After about two weeks, I began to think its critics were right—I felt terrible. General fatigue, local muscle soreness, low energy, constant hunger—I experienced it all. But why? What caused this to happen? Discouraged but also intrigued, I became an even stronger believer in the powerful effect nutrition has on the body. If the pendulum could swing this far to one side, it must be able to swing the other way equally as far.

The resistance from others in the athletic community to a strictly plant-based diet also intrigued me. I was told by several trainers and coaches that I would need to make a decision: I could either eat a plant-based diet *or* I could be an athlete. Being a naturally curious person, I decided to find out for myself: Could I be a top-level athlete on a plant-based diet?

I turned to medical journals, applied dietary studies, and health and nutrition publications to learn more. I developed a good theoretical understanding of the subject, but would such a diet work in practice? It was at this point that I began to experiment, to make myself the test subject of a plant-based diet, with the goal being nothing short of optimal health and vitality.

Knowing that training is little more than breaking down muscle, I figured that what rebuilds that same muscle must be a major factor for recovery and therefore quicker improvement. If I was able to recover from each workout faster, I would be able to schedule them closer together and therefore train more than my competition. I would improve faster. As I suspected, food was the answer—high-quality, nutrient-dense, alkaline-forming, easily digestible food in proper proportions (I learned that last part later). I experimented with a few self-created "performance diets" in an attempt to minimize recovery time between workouts. I began to use my body as a dietary barometer of sorts, based on the knowledge that the sooner I was ready to train again after a workout, the better my diet was. What made some foods speed recovery while others delayed it, sometimes significantly? Nutrition has a dramatic effect on recovery—that was unmistakable. Now I needed to determine what foods were best and why, and what their common denominators were. This would not be an easy task. As with endurance training itself, it could not be rushed. An in-depth experiment of this magnitude would need time. And I made time for it. I began 17 years ago.

Over the course of several years, I started to see a pattern—a series of common denominators began to emerge. The characteristics that rendered some foods highly valuable to the body while others registered as near worthless or actually stress-causing were beginning to present themselves. These former would become the basis for the Thrive Diet.

I then developed a series of test recipes and a week-long meal plan based on foods with the characteristics I found valuable. The result was astounding. Not only did my recovery time plummet but my energy level, strength-to-weight ratio, and endurance shot up. It was several years in the making, but here it was, the basis for the program. Applying the principles, I concocted a blender drink packed with nutrient-dense, plant-based whole foods, which I drank daily.

The year was now 1996 and I was 21. With this program intact, I started training more—because I could. I was recovering at an unprecedented rate. At this point, I realized that my goal of racing Ironman triathlon professionally *was* realistic. Just two years later, in 1998, I began my professional career. The speed at which my body was able to adapt to this type of all-encompassing training was my most impressive achievement. I attribute these exceptionally fast gains to the detailed attention I paid to my diet.

Over the years, the core parameters of the diet have not changed, having withstood the test of time. That's not to say that the diet has not evolved—it has. I've added new foods to the nutrition program once they have passed the recovery test and also been validated by published research.

What I realized next would become one of the most important implications of the diet. That the diet helped speed my recovery was great, but on a broader scale, there was so much more to be realized. Indeed, that recovery time between workouts could be significantly shorter was itself an indication of far more. On the cellular level, this diet was able to speed the renewal of muscle tissue. That meant that following this diet would actually help the body regenerate more frequently, suggesting that it could help reduce biological age. (I discuss this aspect in detail in Chapter 2.) There was more though: A major determinant of rate of recovery is stress level. The more stress placed on the body, the slower recovery will take place. When my external stress stayed at a constant level and the only variable was what I ate, it became clear to me that my plant-based diet helped reduce stress simply through better nutrition. This concept became the premise of the Thrive Diet. In Chapter 1, I expand on this, explaining the different forms of stress.

The implication that this diet could reduce stress was significant. Stress is now understood to be the root cause of many diseases and other health ailments. Obesity, fatigue, poor digestion, and trouble sleeping are often symptoms of stress. Since the average North American is plagued by stress of varying types, the stress-reducing premise of the Thrive Diet is the ideal solution for staying healthy in our modern-day world. This diet was no longer just for high-level athletes—it was suitable for all people, no matter their activity level: By helping reduce nutritional stress, and thereby overall stress, the Thrive Diet is beneficial for everyone. In fact, the Thrive Diet will potentially eliminate up to 40 percent of the total stress on the average North American's body.

I discuss nutritional stress in detail in Chapter 1, but, in short, *nutritional stress* is the term used to describe the body's stress response to food that is void of nutrition and/or foods that require a large amount of energy to digest and assimilate—refined, unnatural ones. Nutritional stress has the same damaging physiological effects as other kinds of stress. With modern-day demands and a diet based on refined foods, the average North American's body is under as much stress as that of a professional endurance athlete. Although the source of stress may be different, the need to curtail the negative effects is the same. Stress may be the cause of many health problems, but the good news is that we have control over what we eat and can prevent and reverse many health problems simply by eating a diet that alleviates nutritional stress. That is exactly what I developed the Thrive Diet to do—to get us healthy at the core.

The Thrive Diet aims to:

- reduce biological age,
- increase life expectancy,
- help reduce body fat and maintain lean muscle,
- increase energy without coffee or sugar,
- increase strength and endurance,
- improve productivity,
- improve mental clarity,
- improve sleep quality,
- reduce sleep requirements,
- improve resistance to infection,
- quicken recovery from exercise,
- reduce or eliminate sugar cravings,
- increase desire to excel.

In addition to the Thrive Diet's health benefits, it's easy on the environment. In Chapter 3 I explain how the diet is structured to use as few resources as possible, making it one of the most environmentally friendly diets possible. Environmental preservation translates into higher quality food, which directly affects those who eat it.

In Chapter 4 I explain the value exercise has on regeneration and renewal. I cover what foods are optimal to fuel a workout and which ones are best to be eaten after exercise for quick recovery. Exercise-specific recipes that I've made for myself for years are included.

Chapter 5 is a list and description of the main foods in the diet, and Chapter 6 is a 12-week meal plan that will help you get started on the Thrive Diet. You may choose to follow the meal plan exactly, or simply use it as a general guideline. Along with soaking and sprouting instructions for seeds, nuts, and legumes, you'll find the recipes for the meal plan in Chapter 7. These include recipes for cereals, energy bars, smoothies, burgers, salads, dressings, and much more.

I have also provided an appendix detailing the vitamins, minerals, and other nutrients and food components involved in a healthy diet, as well as a glossary of terms I use often in the book. The Resources section at the back of the book lists companies that make high-quality base ingredients that you can use to make the Thrive Diet recipes.

With this book as your guide, you will be well on your way to reaping the rewards of higher quality living. By applying the principles of the Thrive Diet, you will create the fundamental foundation of health. No step is too small; each aspect of the diet that you embrace will directly translate into meaningful results. Start slow and build.

one

reduce stress to increase vitality

Stress is something that we are all familiar with—our modern world is a breeding ground for it. Yet, many of us aren't aware of how expansive its reach can be and just how deeply it can affect every aspect of our life. Simply put, stress is anything that causes strain. Mental or physical, and regardless of origin, stress, with its far-reaching consequences, affects everyone in some way. The sources of stress in modern life are many; everything from pollutants in our drinking water and poor nutrition, to relationship concerns and job dissatisfaction, to overexercising or underexercising—all are stressors.

Stress is like fire: When controlled and used for a purpose, it serves us well. Left unbridled, it can consume us. In amounts that our body is capable of adapting to, certain stresses are beneficial. Exercise, for example, is a stress. Exercise and then rest, and your body will grow stronger. However, stress has become, now more than ever, a real threat to our health and livelihood, often overwhelming us and, in some cases, even controlling us.

Located on top of the kidneys, our two adrenals are small triangular glands that play a large role in the body's response to stress. During times of elevated stress, regardless of its source, the body's adrenal glands kick into action, secreting the hormone cortisol into the bloodstream. Cortisol is sometimes referred to as the "stress hormone" for the simple reason that its release is triggered by stress.

Because of the release of cortisol in reaction to the onset of stress, our body actually gains energy. We become more alert, our strength may increase, and we are able to process information more quickly and react slightly faster than usual. This is an innate defense mechanism. Drawing on its primal roots, our body assumes that if it is stressed, it must be in danger. By summoning its hormonal resources to temporarily improve strength and reaction time, the body will improve its odds of getting out of a prehistoric bind—early humans, for instance, would have had increased odds of survival when confronted by a predatory animal. Not enough nutrient-supplying food would have also been perceived as a stress to early humans and therefore a threat to survival. The threat would register, evoking the same hormonal response. Greater strength and more energy would have improved their ability to search for food.

The threats to early humans may have been more immediate threats than ours, yet our stress-response mechanism today remains much the same. In modern Western society, rarely is it put to its original use of self-preservation. Our daily threats pale in comparison to being attacked by an animal or having to scour long and hard for food. But although our threats may be less dire, they are greater in number—far greater—and cumulative. Since our primal response to dealing with threats is outdated, stress slowly eats away at us. In fact, our stress-response mechanism worsens the situation because of its *overreaction*. Wanting to protect us when we are confronted with stress—to get us out of even the slightest bind—our adrenal glands release cortisol to spring us into action. Our adrenal glands are taxed daily, even hourly.

Of course, the amount of cortisol released varies, based on the body's perception of the severity of the stressor. But reacting frequently or overreacting to an event as mundane as working overtime is in itself stressful, and as such, stress-producing. Cortisol will eventually "eat away" at the body by breaking down muscle tissue. And while cortisol stimulates us to deal with an apparent threat, regular stimulation brings about fatigue: Since our adrenal glands were not designed to be used as often as they are today, they become overworked, resulting in exhaustion. Adrenal burnout, as it is commonly referred to, is today a widespread problem.

Many, if not all, of our modern-day health problems are caused by stress. Obesity, fatigue, mental fog, sleep disturbances, digestive problems, prematurely wrinkled skin, depression ... the list goes on. If stress, and therefore cortisol, remains elevated, several problems arise to hamper our body's smooth functioning. One is that the body shifts fuel sources. Instead of burning fat as fuel, a stressed person's system will burn carbohydrate in the form of sugar, and the body begins to store the body fat instead of using it for energy. Stress-free people are fat-burning machines. Stressed people, on the other hand, burn and in turn crave carbohydrates. And cravings themselves are a form of psychological stress, as I discuss later in this chapter.

> Stressed people do not burn body fat as fuel as efficiently as do those who are not stressed.

Stress can also cause hormonal imbalance. When cortisol levels change rapidly, the hormone's symbiotic relationship with other hormones is altered. Hormone imbalance may, for instance, affect electrolyte function, reducing the body's ability to stay adequately hydrated. This results in muscle cramping in the short term and, if neglected, wrinkled and less elastic skin. When the body has difficulty maintaining optimal fluid levels, the delivery of nutrients to its cells is compromised. This leads to a host of problems—basic malnutrition being the most obvious. Even if the diet is ideal, the nutrients are of little use if they don't get distributed. Hormone imbalance can also cause slowed mental ability and impair the delivery of messages from the brain to other parts of the body, slowing movement.

Another health concern that regularly crops up as stress mounts is the inability to sleep soundly. We have all likely had difficulty falling asleep after a traumatic event, or perhaps even after taking on a new, uncertain project at work. As you probably suspected, high cortisol levels are again to blame. And lack of sleep further raises cortisol levels. It's a vicious circle: The body has an increased need for sleep at heightened times of stress yet is unable to get it.

my introduction to stress

I learned a lesson the first year I decided to compete in longer races. It was the spring of 1997. I gradually, but significantly, increased my training mileage, by about 10 percent per week. The first few weeks I didn't experience any problems; everything felt good. But as the months wore on and spring became summer, I found that as my rate of exercise increased, my quality of sleep decreased. This was strange. I had assumed that the more exercise I did, the more tired I would be and the better I would sleep. I continued training as usual. As the weeks passed, the quality of my training declined and I developed a greater appetite.

I was putting my body under a great deal of physical stress. As a result, my cortisol rose to a level that adversely affected my sleep quality. Cortisol levels, if elevated high enough, inhibit the body's ability to slip into the deep sleep state known as delta. It's in the delta phase that the body is best able to restore and regenerate itself. Taking longer to reach delta shortens the time spent in this phase if the total sleep time remains the same. Therefore, to achieve the same restored effect, the body needs to sleep longer.

To maintain the quality of my training sessions, I had to sleep almost an extra hour each night. By doing so, I got my season back on track and was able to retain my desired level of training. At the time, I didn't realize the cause and so treated the symptom, allowing myself to sleep longer. This method worked but, as I understood later, was far from optimal. Reducing the amount of training would also have treated the symptom, but that too was a far from optimal solution. At the time, my nutrition program was adequate but certainly not great. Some of the stress I was experiencing was certainly nutritionally based. Had I nourished my overworked adrenal glands with high-quality whole foods, my sleep quality would have improved enough to get me back on track.

An even more mysterious situation occurred the following year, my second of full-time Ironman training. I was putting in 8- to 10-hour training days, but despite performing 40 hours of exercise per week, I began to slowly accumulate body fat. Not much, about a pound per week, but it was noticeable, and the extra weight was decreasing my strength-to-weight ratio. How could this be? Was I simply eating too much, more than I could burn? Succumbing to this conventional way of thinking, I tried what most people do to lose fat: I cut back on the amount of food I ate. After a few weeks of consuming less, the situation was even worse: I gained fat faster, plus fatigue was now a real concern.

As it turned out, the cause of this fat accumulation was also the cause of the previous year's compromised sleeps: stress. In this case, physical stress—more than my body could deal with. Had I trained the optimal amount, an amount that my body could recover from, I would have remained lean. As I later learned, the amount of training I was doing stressed my body to the brink. The result was that my cortisol levels were chronically elevated for two months—long enough to gain noticeable body fat.

My adrenal glands were exhausted and my hormonal health sharply declined. Unaware of this, I had reduced my nutrient intake at a time when stress on my body was already extremely high, and so exacerbated the problem. Nutritional stress was now again also an issue. Had I eaten nutrient-rich whole foods instead of less food, I would have helped my body recover from the demands of training. In essence, I would have remained leaner by eating more.

Stress, including not being adequately nourished, results in the accumulation of body fat.

My diet at the time consisted primarily of complex carbohydrates, with a modest amount of protein and almost zero fat. A diet rich in essential fatty acids, like those found in whole flaxseed and hemp foods, would have provided the extra fuel my body needed to function more efficiently, thereby reducing stress.

As I found, even physical stress in the form of overexercising can cause fat to accumulate, so it's no wonder that stress from other sources is a catalyst for obesity. The body perceives not eating enough nutrient-rich foods as stressful. So, yes, there are situations when *eating more* will *reduce* your body-fat percentage. The quality of your diet, however, is paramount. The Thrive Diet is based on nutrient-rich whole foods. Their nutritional stress-reduction properties will help you spend more time in the delta phase of sleep and help you achieve an ideal body weight. Eating only nutrient-rich foods will lead to permanent lower body fat.

If your goal is to lose body fat, ask yourself why it is that you have more body fat than you want. Are you overweight because you consume more calories than your body's activity level can utilize? If so, then a reduction in total calories consumed will help. However, if you are one of the many people who have tried a wide array of diets with only marginal success, it's time to get to the root of the problem. The guidelines in this book will help you minimize nutritional stress to optimize health. After that is accomplished, your body fat will decrease. That is, with the Thrive Diet, it is not necessary to specifically target body fat.

the toll of stress

Initially manifesting as fatigue and weight gain, stress, if untreated, can lead to much more serious conditions. Now accepted as one of the leading causes of illness, stress has been shown to precipitate many diseases. The ability to weaken the immune system is one feat stress is renowned for, and compromised immune function leaves the body susceptible to sickness.

Have you ever noticed that when you work to meet a deadline—as the pressure mounts and stress rises—sickness is *least* likely to strike? Then, once you've met the deadline, you get sick. Or perhaps a day or two after a long, taxing race, illness sets in. The body is capable of rising to the occasion in a stressful environment; indeed, the more stress, the better the performance—short term. But when the project is finished and the stress is alleviated, the body *lets* itself get sick. We are equipped with a mechanism that is quite effective at warding off infection until we rest. It assumes that our immune system will be better able to deal with sickness when we are resting and relaxed than if we are in the midst of a pressing time, and it's right. From this, you might conclude that high stress all the time is the solution. Not so. The severity by which the immune system is suppressed is directly linked to the duration and intensity of the stress. Meaning, the longer the body is stressed, the greater is the potential for a big problem.

The body can tolerate only a certain amount of stress; there is a finite amount it can cope with. Strain beyond that point manifests itself in various ways. The first indications that the body is stressed beyond its ability to cope are relatively mild: fatigue, sleep disturbances, and mental fog. If stress overload is more severe, significant weight gain, intense food cravings, and depression become the telltale signs that stress has overwhelmed the system. If these symptoms are not dealt with, if they are allowed to become chronic, the chances of developing a disease such as type II diabetes, fibromyalgia, or even cancer greatly increase.

nutrition and cognitive ability

It continually surprises me how little credence many people place on nutrition's role in achieving and sustaining mental health. As I discuss in Chapter 2, the impact of high-quality food on the reconstruction of cellular tissue cannot be underestimated. The quality of this reconstruction is heavily dependent on the building blocks we make available—as with all other body parts, the brain is sustained and nourished by the food we eat. Constantly orchestrating countless calculations and assessments in just milliseconds, the brain is responsible for keeping us safe. It is in our best interest to keep it healthy.

Amino acids, found in unrefined protein, are our body's prime construction foods. Essential fatty acids are also vital for healthy brain construction and function. Glucose and fructose, two sugars found in fruit, are the brain's preferred source of fuel. I discuss all these nutrients later in the book.

Another important role nutrition plays in brain function involves our blood cells. Our blood cells serve several purposes, including distributing nutrients throughout the body and aiding digestion. Although many parts of the body require blood to function properly, blood is drawn to the part of the body where it is needed most. When we eat poorly digestible refined foods, extra blood is drawn to the stomach to help digestion. Because the blood is drawn away from parts that also require it, other bodily functions are slowed. You may have noticed after eating a large, heavy meal that your energy dwindles, that your body slows down. Try concentrating on something that requires considerable thought—it's difficult. The brain cannot get the blood it needs to function optimally. Not enough blood in the head means not enough nutrients to the brain, and since red blood cells carry oxygen, a heavy meal deprives the brain of oxygen as well. It's no wonder people have trouble concentrating after a big meal. In Spain, it is common to take a nap after lunch. Lunch is that country's heaviest meal of the day. The Spanish don't fight it; they know the body needs to work hard to digest, so they give themselves a break and allow themselves time to recharge. One of the benefits of eating whole, unrefined foods, like those featured in the Thrive Diet, are their low impact on the digestive system and other biological functions. Those who eat according to the Thrive Diet will have a greater ability to think clearly after consuming a meal.

cravings

One reason why people become overweight is because they eat too much of the unhealthy types of fat. Why do people crave fat? Fat helps numb the receptors in the brain that regulate emotional responses; that is, eating foods high in fat will help diminish certain unwanted feelings—at least in the short term. The best way to stop fat cravings is to eliminate the cause of the sadness, and that's easiest done once mental and physical well-being is achieved. The Thrive Diet meal plan will get you on your way.

Too much stress can result in depressed, low moods. In response, the ever resourceful brain attempts to self-medicate. Cravings are the first sign of this. To understand why our brain behaves this way, we again need to look to our primitive roots, to a time when forms of sugar could be found *only* in nutrient-rich fruit. Early humans craved sweet foods, just as we do, yet these cravings were satisfied exclusively by eating fruit. When stress goes up, so does our need for high-quality nutrition. Fruit provided it for early humans: The brain "assumed" that sweet meant nutrition in the form of fruit. However, most sweets that people eat today—in the form of refined carbohydrates and processed sugars—are nutritionally empty.

A sweet tooth also helps us maintain a positive outlook: The modern brain craves sugary or refined starchy foods (those foods whose fiber has been removed and therefore whose sugar component of the carbohydrate is relatively high) because they release serotonin, a chemical found in the brain's pituitary gland. The release of serotonin has a powerful elevating effect on our mood. Continually low levels of serotonin can lead to chronic fatigue and clinical depression. People who have a regular supply of serotonin being released into their bloodstream feel better, and are therefore more productive and feel less stressed, than those with low levels of serotonin. Serotonin is plentiful and free flowing when stress is low; however, as stress rises, serotonin production declines. Cravings for sugary or starchy food are most likely an attempt by the brain to make it "feel" better. This is why such foods are referred to as comfort foods—they are the foods that are craved after a particularly trying day. Ice cream and donuts, which are high in the sugar required to produce the subconsciously desired serotonin hit, are common comfort foods. Giving in to these cravings will satisfy the brain, but this satisfaction is short-lived. And so you eat more serotonin-releasing foods, which eventually leads to more stress, since these refined carbohydrates offer very few nutrients—not having enough nutrients in our diet is a form of nutritional stress and therefore produces a stress response. Simply by having lower levels of cortisol (meaning less stress), the body will naturally produce more serotonin. Natural light and healthy food are the best ways to natural raise serotonin.

When our thoughts are uncontrollably occupied by the perceived need for something, that is a craving. Craving specific foods preoccupies the brain, making it less able to focus on anything else: The mental clutter created by cravings causes the brain to be less functional. Some people even consider cravings mentally unhealthy. Albert Einstein was rumored to have worn the same clothes every day. His reasoning was simple: He didn't want to have to *think* about what to wear. Einstein knew that he needed his brain to focus on his ground-breaking work, not day-to-day living. It has also been reported that, for the same reason, Einstein purposely did not remember his phone number—just more mental clutter.

> Stress and in turn food cravings create mental clutter, decreasing the brain's ability to perform to its full potential.

Having specific food cravings hampers ideas from flowing freely: If these cravings are constantly part of our mental functioning, meaning the brain is focused on getting something at the chemical level, it makes sense that the likelihood of having ideas "just hit us" is reduced. It's like having a radio constantly on—even if it's at low volume, no matter how hard you try, you can't completely tune it out. If free-flowing thoughts cannot coexist with mental clutter, then new ideas, innovations, and ways to solve problems, generated by the subconscious, will not present themselves as readily or manifest as clearly.

The path to an uncluttered mind begins with stress management, and diet is the number one consideration.

types of stress

Many people complain of symptoms of stress, and some even consult a doctor or other practitioner about them. You may notice that your energy level is down, yet you are also having trouble sleeping; that your tolerance is lower—small things irritate you—and you're having trouble making even minor decisions. These are all typical signs of stress. Typically, the advice we receive is to not engage in as many stressful activities—"Don't work as much" or "Slow down and take more time for yourself." Following such advice is one way to reduce stress. However, doing so also reduces productivity, which can actually *contribute* to stress: The last thing a high achiever wants to hear is that he or she should slow down.

It's easy to say, "Reduce the amount of stress in your life and you'll be healthier." While this is generally a true statement, it's too broad. Instead, "select" your stressors; cultivate the beneficial ones and eliminate the unbeneficial. All stressors can be classified into one or more of three categories: uncomplementary, complementary, and production. It is possible to greatly reduce stress and its debilitating effects without reducing productivity; in fact, productivity will *improve* if the right stressors are removed. Energy improvement, ability to recover from exercise quickly, and a healthy body weight are just a few of the benefits of removing uncomplementary stress.

uncomplementary stress

Uncomplementary stress is the term I use to describe anxiety that produces no benefit. This type of stress should be eliminated or at

Breakdown of Stressors

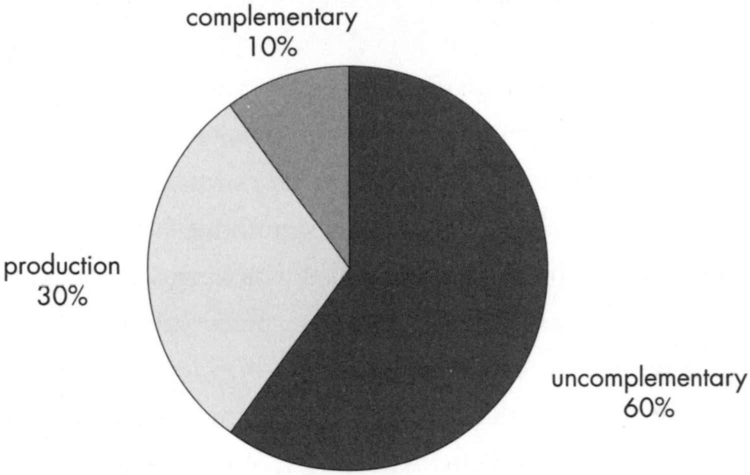

Common Sources of Uncomplementary Stress

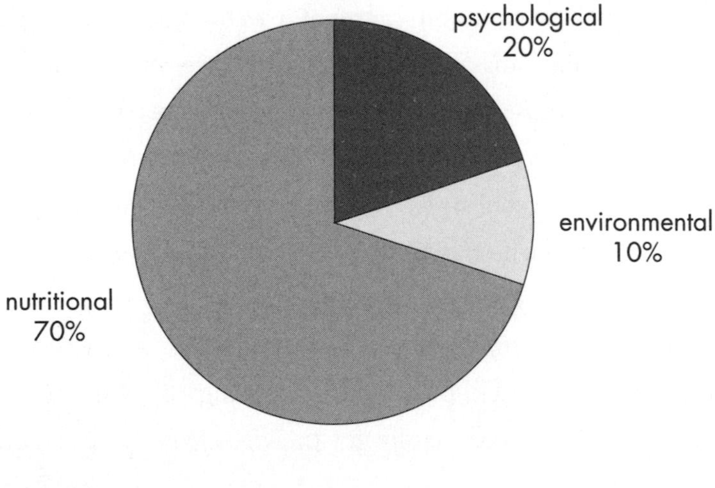

least reduced as much as possible, since there is nothing to be gained by it. A chief goal of the Thrive Diet is to reduce uncomplementary stress.

It's estimated that as much as 60 percent of the average North American's total stress can be categorized as uncomplementary. That's a huge amount, particularly given this stress's debilitating effects, with no payoff to its host. Environmental stress accounts for roughly 10 percent of all uncomplementary stress. Air pollution, on the rise in urban areas especially, is a significant factor in environmental stress: We are breathing air laced with toxins. The abundance of internal combustion engines in vehicles poses the most immediate air-quality threat in urban centers. On a broader scale, inefficient food production and the transportation of this food is the biggest threat to air quality and environmental health as a whole. I discuss food production and the environment in detail in Chapter 3.

Psychological stress accounts for about 20 percent of total uncomplementary stress. This kind of stress is generally self-imposed, and some people are more prone to it than others. Worrying about future events that are in no way controllable, such as the weather, is a mild form of psychological stress. Setting unrealistic goals and then failing to meet them is a common cause of psychological stress. Feeling generally unfulfilled, dissatisfied, or criticized are yet other forms. It's been shown that those who regularly receive unconstructive criticism from a person they care for develop a weakened immune system because of their elevated stress. (Interestingly, criticism received from strangers or people who the recipient of the criticism does not like has little if any effect on immune function.)

Here's another example of psychological stress. A friend recently had the flu. He got sick, he says, from "being stressed and getting rundown." Later he joked that he got the virus from his computer. In effect, that *is* what happened. His computer became contaminated with a virus, which erased the hard drive—and all his files. As you can imagine, my friend experienced psychological stress from this event. The stress weakened his immune system, and his body became vulnerable to infection—in this case, the flu. So, while the computer did not literally pass on its virus, it did have an effect on his immune system, paving the road for a biological viral attack.

Nutritional stress, for the average North American, is by far the greatest source of uncomplementary stress, accounting for approximately 70 percent of it. *Nutritional stress* is a relatively new term. It is simply defined as stress created by food because of its unhealthy properties. This definition is far-reaching, encompassing most food many of us consider staples. And while this definition is accurate, it is not complete—nutritional stress is much more than just unhealthy food. *Not* eating the right foods can cause nutritional stress: Not eating *enough* natural, unprocessed foods rich in vitamins, minerals, enzymes, high-quality protein, fiber, essential fatty acids, antioxidants, and good bacteria (probiotics) is a major source of stress on our bodies. Without these nutritional building blocks, the body lacks the components it needs to regenerate completely and effectively. The result is a weaker, less resilient body and, of course, more stress. The Appendix covers nutrients in detail. I explain why they matter and how you can ensure that your diet is rich in them. I also explain how their inclusion in your diet will dramatically reduce total stress.

> The absence of healthy food in the diet is a form of stress.

Regular consumption of nutrient-dense whole foods supports cellular regeneration, which rebuilds new body tissue. This process is vital for every aspect of health and vitality. Nutrient-dense whole foods are those that have not been refined and stripped of their value during processing. Fresh fruit and vegetables, unrefined hemp, flaxseed, quinoa, sprouted nuts, seeds, certain seaweeds, algae, and some types of grains are all examples of such foods. The whole-food recipes in this book, along with the 12-Week Meal Plan (see page 167), will get you going on making whole foods part of your daily diet.

But let's first get back to that common cause of nutritional stress, the overconsumption of refined food. Much of it is consumed in the form of fast food and convenience food—indeed, prepared meals that need only be warmed in the microwave have gained immensely in popularity as North Americans become increasingly busy. Refined, denatured, or fractionalized, these foods are not naturally complete—parts have been removed during processing. White bread is a good example. White flour is made from wheat that has had the germ—the fiber- and mineral-dense part of the wheat—removed from the grain, leaving it nutritionally void. Unlike whole foods, refined foods offer little in the way of nutritional value; they are often simply empty calories. Usually high in refined carbohydrate and harmful types of fat, refined food has no place in the Thrive Diet.

The regular consumption of processed food has been linked to numerous cases of compromised health. The typical North American diet, for instance, has been linked to the development of food sensitivities and food allergies. It has also been shown that many allergies precipitate cravings, making "standard" foods harder to eliminate from the diet. Over time, these eating habits wear down the body's endocrine system, the glandular system that secretes hormones into the bloodstream to regulate bodily functions, and, in turn, our organs' ability to function efficiently. Nutrient deficiencies develop and premature signs of aging reveal themselves. General muscle stiffness and lethargy are sure to follow, and sickness is more likely. Often shrugged off as part of the aging process, symptoms such as these are *not* natural in a middle-aged person: They are a direct result of stress, most of it nutritional. The slowing rate at which the body regenerates at a cellular level is biological aging; the speed at which *that* transpires, however, depends on diet. Combining the destructive nature of a largely refined-food diet with other common stressors and allowing these stressors to continue to the point at which they are chronic paves the way for many ailments—high blood pressure, blood sugar control problems, and elevated blood fats such as cholesterol among them. The immune system will become severely compromised, and this will likely lead to recurrent infections and serious conditions such as chronic fatigue syndrome or fibromyalgia.

In addition to its negative physical effects, uncomplementary stress has been shown to have a significant adverse effect on the psyche and motivation. Scientists now believe that will power is finite; its supply can become exhausted at the hands of excess stress, most notably uncomplementary stress. A person's desire to achieve is closely tied to stress level. That came as a surprise to me. I had always thought that motivation was simply a personality trait—that a person either did or didn't have drive. While personality is a factor, it now seems that there is more to it than that. Regardless of the desire to excel, if a person is forced to deal with mounting stress, that stress can cause motivation to flicker or extinguish altogether.

To use an analogy of a car, will power is burned like fuel. As gasoline is to the internal combustion engine, will power is to stress. Each time the car meets a headwind, it burns more fuel. The greater the resistance, the greater the fuel consumption. If a person is dissatisfied with her workplace—the hours, the lack of aptitude required, and the paycheck all become a source of discontentment. She will be required to "burn" will power to cope with her situation. Having to push herself to get through each workday, she will arrive home, her motivation exhausted. Even minor challenges will appear great. It's important to understand this. Many people believe that those who have trouble obtaining their goals are lazy or simply not motivated. Yet, it might well be that stress is extinguishing their drive; it is stress that is standing between them and their goals, not lack of ability or fortitude.

I can't overemphasize the importance of enjoying your livelihood: You can't be discontent for that many hours of each day and expect to be healthy in other aspects of your life. Even if only subconsciously, your determination will be eroded and making changes, even those as simple as dietary ones, will be a challenge. The Thrive Diet requires fewer biological resources—less expenditure of energy digesting—and therefore won't place stress on the body. Plus, it is highly nourishing, which is itself a stress-reducing quality. Less uncomplementary stress translates into more drive, and drive is the catalyst for change. Following the dietary principles of the Thrive Diet will have a snowball effect: The body will begin to adapt to the changes, thereby reducing its stress level, which in turn will pave the way for even greater progress.

Uncomplementary stress depletes motivation, making even small challenges seem daunting.

Food production is also a big culprit in nutritional stress. Conventional farming involves the ongoing use of chemical fertilizers, herbicides, and pesticides on food crops. Unlike organic farming, conventional farming employs chemical dustings to discourage insects and rodents from eating the crops. If a pest deterrent—poison—is sprayed on both the crops and the soil, there is a good chance it will find its way into our food. Designed to kill small pests, pesticides when consumed by humans can at the very least cause a reaction from the immune system as it attempts to defend the body.

People with suppressed immune function will likely experience even more of an impact, sometimes succumbing to sickness.

Ground water seepage is a concern, too. Will the pesticides, having made their way into the soil, eventually end up in the water supply? According to some experts, this is exactly what is happening: Municipal drinking water supplies have tested positive for agricultural runoff. Drinking water that contains pesticides will obviously have an adverse effect on our immune system and health.

As destructive and prevalent as uncomplementary stress is, its positive aspect is that we have control over it. Understand it and take steps to eliminate it, with the Thrive Diet as your guide.

complementary stress

I call the right amount of stress to stimulate renewal and instigate growth within the body *complementary stress*. Exercise is a form of complementary stress. Essentially nothing more than breaking down muscle tissue, exercise is the best way to stimulate regeneration of the cells.

Have you ever noticed that those who exercise regularly look younger than those who don't? Although we have no control over our chronological age, our biological age is within our control. Biological age refers to the time that has passed since body cells last regenerated. When exercised, the body must regenerate its cells more rapidly than when idle. Depending on activity level, six to eight months from now our bodies will have regenerated nearly 100 percent of their tissue at the cellular level. This new tissue will literally be made up of what we eat between now and then. The body of an active person is forced to regenerate rapidly; therefore, it consists of more recently produced—younger—cells, making for a younger body.

Exercise is also complementary in its ability to raise the body's tolerance to physical activity. If a person exercises regularly and is in fair shape, everyday physical activities will not produce a stress response. This is significant. Here's why. If someone who exercises regularly walks up a few flights of stairs, for example, the strain from doing so will be far below what the body is accustomed to enduring in a workout. The strain on the body from ascending the stairs will not even be noticeable, meaning no stress response. Cortisol, the body's stress-fighting hormone, will not rise, and the immune system will not in turn decline. A fit person who engages in even minor physical activity will be less likely to succumb to ailments than will a person who does not exercise consistently.

Similarly, people who jog on a regular basis experience no stress response from walking and very little from running slowly. Conversely, the body of a person who does not exercise regularly will perceive minor physical activity as a strain, and this will trigger a stress response. This is something to be mindful of when beginning an exercise program. Until the body has adapted to the higher level of stress, the immune system will be vulnerable. (Avoiding contact with people who have a virus until your body has adjusted to the higher level of exercise is a good idea.)

The right balance of exercise strengthens us, both mentally and physically. Exercising the optimal amount (which is determined by your ability to recover and deal with other stresses) will strengthen the body as a whole. Gains include improved muscle tone, a reduction in body fat, increased strength-to-weight ratio, improved immune function, clearer thinking, and better sleep quality. Exercise creates a complementary circle: It activates the natural healing and regeneration process of the body.

Ironically, complementary stress can arise when uncomplementary stress is no longer tolerable and so positive change is instigated. When stress reaches a point that it can no longer be suppressed, dealt with, or tolerated, it begins to motivate and prompt action; change *must* transpire. Mild dissatisfaction in the workplace, for example, is among the least healthy of long-term situations. Since it is usually bearable on a day-to-day basis, it is often tolerated—sometimes for years. The cumulative effect of this daily mild discontent is stress-related health problems. However, when job dissatisfaction reaches the point at which it is no longer tolerable, action for change *will* occur. Like a slow leak in a car tire, you may tolerate it, refilling the tire with air as needed. Yet, if the tire were to rip open, making driving impossible, you would change it immediately. Many people put up with things that are unpleasant but tolerable, rather than changing them; their situation needs to become unbearable before they take action. So, in effect, an unbearable job is better than one that is simply dissatisfying, since it will be the catalyst for change.

production stress

Production stress is the stress created when you strive to achieve a goal. Ranging from physically demanding training sessions for an athletic competition or working overtime on an important project to sorting out family problems or taking a calculated risk, production stress is not something to shy away from. Sometimes referred to as the "high achiever's syndrome," production stress, as its name implies, is an unavoidable by-product of a productive life, a necessary part of modern-day success.

My production stress, when racing Ironman triathlons professionally, was physical—it was the at-times-unhealthy amount of exercise that I had to do in order to improve as an athlete. This physical production stress differed from complementary stress in the sense that it was actually in excess of what was healthy. The 35 hours of weekly training required to be competitive takes its toll on the body. Before I could undertake this type of training, I had to build a platform of optimal health to support it. However, during that intense training, it was no longer about health but performance—such is the nature of competitive sports. Although the immune system weakens and cortisol levels rise, to engage in this kind of activity for short periods has a payoff. In my case, it was greatly increased fitness and the ability to race at a high level. I had to, however, reduce all other stressors as much as possible to accommodate the augmented physical strain that came with the training load. And, as you may have guessed by now, reducing nutritional stress was the biggest component.

But, as I've mentioned, production stress is not limited to the physical. Working tirelessly on a sedentary project can be equally demanding and equally rewarding. Production stress can be viewed simply as achieving. For example, working tirelessly on a project at work or school can undoubtedly be a strain, yet on completion, you have a product. Whether a tangible one as a result of work or simply more knowledge from study, it is something that you did not have before you *worked* for it. Whatever the circumstances, bringing on production stress by way of striving to achieve something and getting rid of the uncomplementary stress is a sound strategy that I recommend to anyone.

A certain amount of stress is an inevitable component of achievement.

stimulation

One type of stress can be categorized either as production or uncomplementary stress, depending on how it is used. It is stimulation. Whether for work, school, sport, or any other activity, it is sometimes in our best interest to summon energy through stimulation. When the adrenal glands are stimulated in order to achieve something that could not be done, or done as well, without this stimulation, the stress that results can be classified as production stress.

Here's an example of a sensible way to use stimulation as production stress. An athlete who has recalibrated his diet (I explain how to do this in Chapter 2) by eating a clean diet and abstaining from stimulating foods such as refined sugar and coffee drinks a cup of yerba maté (a South American herb) tea before a race. The caffeine in the yerba maté will stimulate his adrenal glands, improving his endurance and helping him achieve a better performance than he might otherwise achieve. This will also bring about greater fatigue within a day or two, and that's fine. At the time of the race, the athlete simply borrowed energy from the future to fuel his performance. Extra fatigue a day or two later will be a small price to pay for his performance. The same holds true for those trying to get more done at work. Stimulation can enable them to achieve more in the short term.

However, if this borrowing strategy is used too often, it will lose its effectiveness and simply become another form of uncomplementary stress. To be effective, the strategy can be used only a few times a month, once a week at most, for those times when a boost would really be beneficial. Ideally, you would rarely, if ever, need it; the Thrive Diet is structured in such a way that there will be no desire or need to borrow energy.

If stimulation is used when it will not help you achieve something of value, it is an uncomplementary stress. I consider coffee drinking an uncomplementary stress. I view it as a form of credit, similar to shopping with a credit card. You get energy now that you don't actually have, but you pay for it later—when the "bill," or fatigue, hits. (Simply drinking more coffee to put off the inevitable is like paying off one credit card with another: It will catch up with you sooner or later.) You'll most likely pay a high interest rate as well, needing more time to recover than if that energy had not been borrowed in the first place. This is the beginning of a vicious circle. In the next chapter, I provide strategies to recalibrate the body, and in doing so, get maximum energy simply from eating natural food.

At a Glance

- Stress is the root cause of most ailments, both minor and major, in the North American population.
- About 40 percent of the average North American's total stress can be attributed to diet.
- Excessive stress can have a negative psychological effect and can be responsible for specific food cravings and mental clutter.
- Improved diet is the number one way to reduce overall stress.
- Complementary stress can build physical strength and improve motivation.
- Once diet is improved, production stress can be embraced, and productivity will therefore be enhanced.

two

understanding the thrive diet

The Thrive Diet is basic, and its parameters are simple. As you've just learned, uncomplementary stress is the biggest threat to our well-being. Unfortunately, its avoidance is near impossible in Western society. However, we do have the ability to take our health into our own hands and by doing so live a high-energy, sickness-free, rewarding life.

The word *health* is thrown around quite freely these days. However, the word really does embrace all that we physiologically and psychologically can aspire to. If we all had a high level of health, we would all be at our ideal body weight, none of us would have food cravings, we would all sleep soundly, we wouldn't rely on stimulating foods to give us energy, and we would always be able to think clearly and rationally. Yet, few of us are in this situation. One of the reasons is because we often treat the symptoms of each ailment as it crops up, while ignoring its cause.

Simply put, the Thrive Diet is about getting to the root of the matter. Symptom-treating programs have risen in popularity over the past several years because of the speed at which results can be seen, and treating symptoms has become the excepted approach for many. While it's true that short-term results can be achieved by dealing merely with the symptoms, long-term sustainable satisfaction is rarely if ever achieved. The Thrive Diet will likely not produce noticeable result as quickly as some symptom-treating methods. However, the Thrive Diet *is* a platform for long-term success. It is a healthy, well-balanced diet, with a focus on long-term sustainability. Those who eat a healthier diet are healthier: They are close to their ideal body weight, they have more energy and more motivation, and, quite simply, they get more out of life.

The Thrive Diet treats the root cause of the problem.

Results that you can expect from the Thrive Diet include:

- improved ability to burn body fat as energy,
- better sleep quality, therefore less needed,
- elimination of junk-food cravings,
- reduced body fat,
- less joint inflammation,
- improved mental clarity,
- eliminated need to rely on stimulants for energy,
- improved ability to build lean muscle tissue,
- quick recovery from exercise,
- reduced cholesterol level,
- stronger bones,
- better skin quality.

high net-gain nutrition is the key

The first and most general guideline of the Thrive Diet is to make high net-gain foods a cornerstone of your diet. The *net gain* of food is the term I use to describe the energy and usable sustenance that our body is left with once the food has been digested and assimilated. The body gets energy from food by way of nutrients. The more energy the body must expend to digest, assimilate, and utilize the nutrients in the food we give it, the less energy we are left with. As I mentioned earlier, the Thrive Diet was designed to reduce stress. For nutritional stress to be minimized, efficiency of digestion and nutrient assimilation must be maximized. Essentially, what high net-gain eating does is eliminate excess work for the body. And as you know, work without benefit equals uncomplementary stress.

Unfortunately, most foods in the average North American's diet require almost as much energy to assimilate as they contain. They therefore have an extremely low net gain. The nutritional value of food stated on the food packaging label refers to what is in the food—not what the body actually gets from it. The digestion process requires energy, a large portion of which is expelled as heat. People who eat a standard North American diet, one that includes many processed foods, burn a significant amount of energy digesting it. Similar to an incandescent light bulb that throws off heat inadvertently when producing light, the substantial amount of heat created and expelled during digestion translates into a significant net energy loss. Bodies that constantly operate at a high temperature are simply not operating efficiently. Energy used digesting the food is turned into heat that is then expelled into the environment. As heat escapes the body, so does energy. Had energy not been lost through this process—if it had been conserved through greater digestive efficacy—it might have been used as fuel for other body functions or fabrication of new cellular tissue.

Because high net-gain foods are more easily digested, you may notice that your core body temperature drops slightly when you follow the Thrive Diet. During the colder winter months, in particular, this will be noticeable. While much healthier and a testament to an efficient body, a lower temperature may take getting used to.

We can all benefit significantly from a body that retains energy by operating more efficiently, and the advantage for athletes is particularly great. Starting with a lower core temperature provides a larger "window" in which to operate. When physical intensity rises, so too does body temperature. By starting at a lower point, the athlete will be able to generate a greater intensity before reaching the maximum temperature that the body can efficiently function under. That is, a lower operating temperature translates into the ability to perform more work before experiencing fatigue. Here's an example: If two runners were running side by side and one's core temperature was a degree lower than the other's, she would be farther from her body's maximum temperature. This would allow her to speed up, running ahead of the other runner while exerting no more effort. Also, being farther from maximum temperature means that her body, and therefore heart, do not have to work as hard, allowing her heart rate to stay lower. A lower heart rate means that less energy is being expended to maintain physical workload, and therefore her endurance is improved.

I am often asked how I am able to gain and maintain strength and lean muscle, and have an abundance of energy for high-performance training, while eating fewer calories than most people. One of the most important factors is that I select food with the net-gain concept in mind rather than by the conventional calorie-counting method. Let's consider white bread. In the old days, when dining out, I would wolf down the French bread typically served before the meal. My stomach would be physically full, yet I would still be hungry. Since white bread is void of any useful nutrients, my body wanted me to continue eating despite that I felt full. To digest, assimilate, and then eliminate the white bread requires a large energy expenditure. The net energy gain from it is very low. If the bread is buttered or if a spread containing trans fat is added, the result can be a net energy loss.

In today's hectic, fast-paced world, we are inundated with nutrient-deficient foods. Consumed mostly for convenience sake, processed and refined foods have led us to a decline in health and to elevated medical costs. Because of their absence of usable nutrients, we find we have to consume more and more of these foods to fill ourselves up. Thanks to their high refined sugar and calorie counts, we have become an obese, energy-depleted society.

A calorie is defined as a measure of food energy. It might seem logical, then, to assume that the more calories consumed, the more energy our body is supplied with. Of course, we know this is not the case, otherwise people with the highest energy would be those who eat at fast food restaurants. By simply consuming more calories, we are not guaranteed more energy. Many conventional nutrition books would have us believe that if we expend a certain amount of energy, it can be quantified and replaced. They suggest that by simply adhering to calorie counts, with no consideration of other factors, we can accurately gauge the amount of food we need to consume to maintain low body weight and high energy. But it doesn't work that way.

Several years ago, before I had created the Thrive Diet, I did try to gauge my caloric intake requirements based on my activity level and body weight. Eating about 8000 calories on heavy training days, the number of calories I determined I required, I usually needed a rest day soon afterward. I realize now that a large part of my need for the rest day was not so much to recover from the energy expended during training as to recover from the energy expended digesting all that food. I ate lots of starchy, high-carbohydrate foods such as white pasta and bread. Roasted nuts, usually in the form of peanut butter, was also a large part of my high-calorie yet low-nutrient diet. These are hard for the body to digest and assimilate and have little to offer in terms of nutrients, and so I was robbing myself of energy with every bite.

I also discovered that there were several other ways in which standard foods cause the body to be in a constant state of elevated stress. Fortunately, as many problems as conventional foods can cause, high net-gain foods can alleviate.

I found that by consuming more easily assimilated foods, I could conserve a large amount of energy, therefore reducing stress in my body. There are two main reasons for this. First, foods in their natural, nutrient-dense state can be digested and assimilated with less energy expenditure than processed, refined foods. Second, when more nutrient-rich foods are present in the diet, the body does not have to eat as much as if it were fed less nutrient-rich foods. In addition, when the body is fed the nutrients it needs, the brain turns off the hunger signal. And so, the need to continually consume, a state many people who subsist on a refined-food diet experience, ceases, and not as much needs to be eaten and digested. And since, as I noted above, the digestion and assimilation process for many processed foods is an exceptionally large energy draw, cutting out such foods will immediately translate into a net-energy surplus, meaning more usable energy. And with this extra energy, the body will likely choose to improve immune function and quicken restoration of cells damaged by stress—essentially, anti-aging activities.

Once I realized the value in nutrient density, assimilation, and absorption of food, I began eating in terms of net gain, rather than to calorie-consumption guidelines. I focused on consuming nutrient-dense, easily assimilated foods. As a result, my recovery rate has significantly improved. I no longer need an extra day to recover from eating copious amounts of conventional food. Enhanced by increased efficacy, my body now pools its retained energy resources to more quickly recover from muscle damage associated with training. Today, I consume about 30 percent fewer calories than I did just two years ago, yet I have more energy—by means of conservation, rather than consumption.

Instead of feasting on refined foods, I now consume whole foods almost exclusively. Raw, alkalizing, enzyme-intact foods have become the foundation of my diet. Switching my main carbohydrate source from refined starches to whole fruits and vegetables was my starting point. In doing so, the majority of my energy needs, once obtained primarily from carbohydrate, are now being met by a wide variety of fruit, complemented by pseudograins. Although commonly referred to as a grain, pseudograins are actually seeds. Higher in protein, fiber, and trace minerals than grains, pseudograins are also gluten-free. The ones I use most frequently in my recipes are amaranth, buckwheat, and quinoa.

The consumption of nutrient-dense foods reduces the stress response and allows the body to conserve energy, to be used as fuel and building blocks.

And so, as I said earlier, the cornerstone of the Thrive Diet is high net-gain foods. It's that simple. By eating more high net-gain foods, your energy will rise, body fat will decrease, mental clarity will be enhanced, and cravings for refined foods will fade. The Thrive Diet is designed to be easy to follow and stick to. I believe that strictly imposed parameters, though they may work for some people in the short term, are not the way to long-term success. I find that they often create more stress, thereby reducing the effectiveness of the program. The Thrive Diet is a way of life, more of a philosophy than a program. To me, blindly following a strict program is not a mentally healthy way to seek health. I created the Thrive Diet to serve as a platform on which self-reliance can be built.

So what exactly constitutes high net-gain foods? The Thrive Diet of high net-gain foods is based on the following guiding principles. Eat primarily foods that are—

- raw or cooked at low temperature,
- naturally alkaline-forming foods to pH balance the body (discussed later in this chapter, on page 47),
- high in nutrients the body can use without having to convert them (I call this one-step nutrition),
- nutrient-dense whole foods,
- vitamin- and mineral-rich, from whole-food sources,
- non-stimulating, to recalibrate the body and eliminate biological debt.

The tiers of the Thrive Diet pyramid show the suggested ratio of each food group in the daily diet. This is not meant to suggest that

The Thrive Diet Pyramid

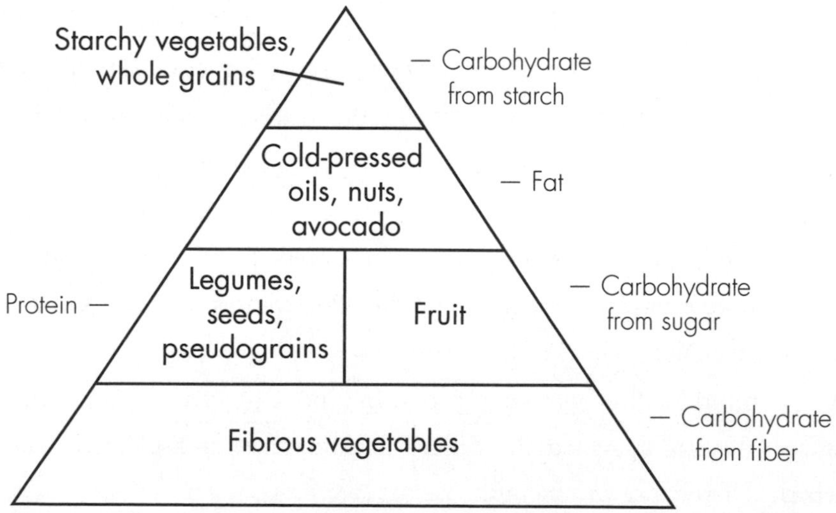

foods higher on the pyramid are of any less value than those on the bottom. The different levels combine to deliver a balance of premium nutrition, each group instrumental in the whole. By volume, the diet consists roughly of 45 percent fibrous vegetables; 20 percent fruit; 20 percent legumes, seeds, and pseudograins; 10 percent cold-pressed oils, nuts, and avocado; and 5 percent starchy vegetables and whole grains.

The pyramid is a guide only. You do not need to strictly adhere to it on a daily basis to gain the benefits of the Thrive Diet. However, longer periods should reflect the proportions illustrated in the pyramid. For example, some snacks might include only one of the food groups—say, fruit; even your diet on an entire day may be outside the guidelines. That's fine, as long as over the course of a week or so, the diet shapes up to closely resemble the pyramid.

The Thrive Diet food pyramid is based on fiber-rich carbohydrate. Vegetables constitute the base of the pyramid. With an emphasis on leafy green vegetables and colorful vegetables, this tier offers lots of variety. In addition to supplying fibrous carbohydrate, foods in this tier are a rich source of vitamins, minerals, and phytonutrients. These foods include:

Beets
Bell peppers
Carrots
Celery
Cucumbers
Daikon
Jicama (a legume, though its nutritional makeup resembles more closely that of a non-sweet fruit)

Leafy greens:
- Arugula
- Baby red chard
- Baby spinach
- Beet greens
- Butter lettuce
- Collard greens
- Dandelion greens
- Dinosaur kale
- Frisée
- Gold chard

- Green chard
- Green curly kale
- Green leaf lettuce
- Green oak leaf lettuce
- Kale
- Lollo rosa
- Mâche
- Mizuna
- Mustard greens
- Nagoya
- Pea greens
- Radicchio
- Red Belgian endive
- Red leaf lettuce
- Red mustard
- Red oak leaf lettuce
- Red peacock
- Red romaine lettuce
- Red Russian kale
- Romaine lettuce
- Ruby chard
- Spinach
- Swiss chard
- Tango
- Tat soi
- White nagoya
- White peacock

Sea vegetables:

- Agar
- Arame
- Dulse
- Kombu
- Wakame

Squash

Tomatoes

Zucchini

The second tier of the pyramid comprises two sections. The first delivers primarily protein. Legumes, seeds, and pseudograins, this section is broader than it may at first appear. It includes:

Legumes, all kinds:

- Beans: adzuki, black, fava, kidney
- Lentils: brown, green, red
- Peas: black-eyed, green, yellow

Pseudograins:

- Amaranth
- Buckwheat
- Quinoa
- Wild rice

Seeds, all kinds:

- Flaxseed
- Hemp
- Sesame
- White chia

Sprouts, all kinds:

- All legumes and seeds listed above, sprouted
- Alfalfa
- Broccoli
- Onion

The second section of this tier consists of simple carbohydrate in the form of fruit, rich in antioxidants. It includes:

Apples
Apricots
Bananas
Berries (blackberries, blueberries, cranberries, raspberries, strawberries)
Cherries
Dates
Dragon fruit
Figs
Grapefruit
Grapes
Kiwis
Mangos
Melons (cantaloupe, honeydew, watermelon)
Nectarines
Oranges
Papayas
Peaches
Pears
Pineapples
Plums
Pomegranates

The pyramid's third tier is made up of high-quality fats, all in the health-promoting form of fatty acids, including essential fatty acids. It includes:

Avocado
Coconut: meat and milk
Raw nuts:
- Brazil nuts
- Cashews
- Hazelnuts
- Pecans
- Pine nuts
- Pistachios
- Walnuts

Raw (unrefined) cold-pressed oils:
- Coconut
- Flaxseed
- Green tea seed
- Hemp seed
- Olive, extra-virgin
- Pumpkin seed

The final tier consists of starches, primarily from whole unmodified grains and starchy vegetables. It includes:

New potatoes
Parsnips
Squash
Sweet potatoes
Turnips
Whole grains:
  Barley
  Bulgur wheat
  Oats
  Rice
  Rye
  Spelt
Yams

raw and low-temperature cooked foods

enzyme enhancement

Food that has not been heated above about 118 degrees Fahrenheit is considered to be raw. High-temperature cooking and processing of food destroys the enzymes and nutrients that allow the food to be efficiently digested. Therefore, before the body can make use of cooked food, it must produce enzymes to aid in the digestion process. That takes work—an energy draw that creates a nominal amount of stress.

One of the least appreciated yet most important components of our diet, enzymes are vital to achieving optimal health. An absence of enzymes in your diet can result in the same sickness and disease associated with malnutrition, even if your diet is otherwise healthy. Without enzymes, food cannot be turned into usable fuel for the body. As with hormones, enzyme production in the body diminishes with age, leaving us reliant on diet to provide them.

In the distant past, that was of little concern, as enzymes were plentiful in food. But today enzymes are not so abundant in our foods. As our fresh whole-food choices dwindle, making way for highly refined, processed options, enzymes in our foods diminish. Meanwhile, our ailments are on the rise. Coincidence? Probably not. I believe poor dietary habits and stress are again at the root of the problem. Poor diet depletes our system: The digestion of starchy, sugary, and fatty foods is a major draw on body-produced enzymes, further diminishing our precious supply.

Plant foods have several advantages, including easy digestibility and bioavailability (the rate at which the food is absorbed by the body and exerts an effect). Fatigue, bloating, cramping, and an upset stomach can often be attributed to poor digestion. Many whole plant foods have enzymes that facilitate quick and efficient digestion. The quicker nutrients are extracted from the food, the sooner the food can be eliminated—a key factor in optimal health. As well, insoluble fibrous plant matter (discussed in Chapter 5) speeds waste through our system, reducing the risk of toxins settling in the colon and then spreading throughout the body.

Enzyme-rich foods help ensure the body makes use of the nutrients in the food.

There is some evidence to suggest that consuming too many processed, cooked foods for several years exhausts the body's enzyme-producing glands, resulting in poor digestion and assimilation of food later in life. This is one possible reason for the rapidity of signs of aging and disease—food is no longer nourishing the body the way it once did, simply because it's not being digested the way it once was.

Stress also destroys enzymes. Stress damages cells that enzymes in part are required to reconstruct. But stress also inhibits the body's ability to produce enzymes, creating a catch-22 situation. Let's look at an example: Pollutants in the air are a draw on the immune system and enzymes are called upon to fortify it, yet this environmental stress is reducing the body's ability to produce the needed enzymes.

The speed and quality of cell reconstruction after exercise depend in part on the body's enzyme levels. If the body does not have enough enzymes to draw on, the reconstructive process will slow, speeding signs of aging. Low enzymatic levels, due partly to stress, slow the repair of stress-related damage, using up more energy over the course of more time. That means that more stress will be created over that period than if the body had the enzymes to speed the recovery in the first place. Since it's a stress, this in turn can lower enzyme levels, creating a vicious circle. Enzymes are a vital part of the regeneration process, which in turn is part of the anti-aging process.

For enzyme health, it would ideal for all of us to eat only raw, organic food the day it's harvested, not be exposed to any environmental pollutants, and to live a stress-free life. Obviously, this is not realistic. But we *can* enhance our enzyme intake and production. Since raw foods have enzymes still intact, they are a vital component of a healthy diet. The Thrive Diet is built on a platform of enzyme-rich foods. Those who follow the diet will simply build and maintain healthy levels of enzymes with no additional effort. Consuming a daily dose of raw foods, reducing uncomplementary stress through proper nutrition, and avoiding enzyme-depleting foods such as starchy and deep-fried products are all important principles of the diet.

inflammation reduction

Food cooked at a high temperature can also cause inflammation in the body. As well as destroying enzymes and converting essential fatty acids into trans fats (a dangerous compound that I discuss in detail in Chapter 5, page 143), high-temperature cooking creates advanced glycation end products, or AGEs. The body perceives AGEs as invaders and so its immune cells try to break down the AGEs by secreting large amounts of inflammatory agents. If this natural process is called on too often, the result will likely be diseases commonly associated with old age but which actually have more to do with toxins created by high-temperature cooking. Less elastic skin, arthritis, poorer memory, joint pain, and even heart conditions are often attributable to inflamed tissue.

alkaline-forming foods to pH balance the body

The balance of acid and alkaline within the body is referred to as pH (meaning "potential of hydrogen"), and measured on a scale ranging from pH 1 (the most acidic) to pH 14 (the most alkaline). A neutral or good pH balance is 7.35; maintaining this balance is vital. If the body's pH drops, meaning our body has become too acidic, the likelihood of ailments rises sharply. An acidic environment within the body negatively affects health at the cellular level. It is not possible to be truly healthy when the body is in a constant state of acidosis (characterized by excessively high acid levels). People with an acidic environment within their body are also prone to fatigue: Since acidity is a stressor, cortisol levels rise, impairing sleep. The consumption of acid-forming foods is the number one cause of an overly acidic system, and the overconsumption of acid-forming foods plays a significant role in one of North America's largest health problems—excessive weight.

Since our body is equipped with buffering capabilities, our blood pH will vary to only a small degree, regardless of diet. The body's ability to cope is a testament to how resourceful it is. Yet, the systems that are recruited to facilitate this buffering use energy and can become strained, and if prolonged, will result in significant stress to the systems, causing immune function to falter and effectively opening the door to a host of diseases.

Low-grade metabolic acidosis—when cells remain in an overly acidic state because of too many acid-forming foods being eaten or a high-stress lifestyle in general—is believed to be a leading cause of several health concerns, including the development of kidney stones, loss of bone mass, and the reduction of growth hormone levels, resulting in loss of lean muscle mass and increase of body fat. Low-grade metabolic acidosis affects the body at a cellular level and is responsible for an increase of free radicals and a decrease in the production of cellular energy. In addition to these serious concerns, viruses and bacteria are able to thrive in an acidic body, again possibly leading to numerous diseases. Interestingly, it is impossible for cancer to develop in an alkaline environment; this shows the importance of alkalinity in disease prevention.

An acidic body can lead to a plethora of health problems, including obesity and serious disease.

So what can we do to prevent all this? The answer is to consume more alkaline-forming foods and fewer acid-forming ones. One factor that significantly raises the pH of food, and in turn the body, is chlorophyll content.

Responsible for giving plants their green pigment, chlorophyll is often referred to as the blood of plants. The botanical equivalent to hemoglobin in human blood, chlorophyll synthesizes energy. Chlorophyll converts the sun's energy that has been absorbed by the plant into carbohydrate. Known as photosynthesis, this process is responsible for life on earth. Since animals and humans eat plants, we too get our energy from the sun, plants being the conduit. Chlorophyll is prized for its ability to cleanse our blood by helping remove toxins deposited by dietary and environmental sources. Chlorophyll is also linked to the body's production of red blood cells, making daily consumption of chlorophyll-rich foods important for ensuring the body's constant cell regeneration and improving oxygen transport in the body and therefore energy levels. Optimizing the body's regeneration of blood cells will also contribute to peak athletic performance.

Although some foods test as acidic, they produce an alkalizing effect once digested. Citrus fruit and balsamic and apple cider vinegar are all acidic, but when consumed, they become highly alkaline-forming. Here's a list of the effect certain foods have on the body once digested.

pH EFFECT OF SELECTED THRIVE DIET FOODS

foods	highly alkaline-forming	alkaline-forming	neutral	slightly acid-forming
vegetables	Asparagus	Squash		
	Beets	Sweet potatoes		
	Bell peppers	Yams		
	Broccoli			
	Carrots			
	Cauliflower			
	Celery			
	Chicory			
	Cucumbers			
	Dill			
	Dulse			
	Green beans			
	Leeks			
	Mixed greens (all leafy greens)			
	Onion			
	Parsley			
	Parsnips			
	Peas			
	Sea vegetables			
	Sprouts (all)			
	Zucchini			
pseudograins		Amaranth		
		Buckwheat		
		Millet		
		Quinoa		
		Wild rice		

pH EFFECT OF SELECTED THRIVE DIET FOODS

foods	highly alkaline-forming	alkaline-forming	neutral	slightly acid-forming
legumes				Adzuki beans
				Black beans
				Black-eyed peas
				Chickpeas
				Lentils
seeds		Sesame	Flax	Pumpkin
			Hemp	Sunflower
			White chia	
fruit	Grapefruit	Apples		
	Lemons	Avocados		
	Limes	Bananas		
	Mangos	Berries (most)		
	Melons (most)	Cantaloupe		
	Papayas	Cherries		
		Dates		
		Figs		
		Grapes		
		Nectarines		
		Oranges		
		Peaches		
		Pears		
		Persimmons		
		Pineapple		
		Pomegranates		
oils		Flaxseed	Coconut	
		Hemp		
		Pumpkin seed		
nuts		Almonds	Macadamia	
		Coconut	Walnuts	
grains				Brown rice
				Oats
				Spelt
flours			Buckwheat	Chickpea
				Hemp
sweeteners	Stevia		Agave nectar	

pH EFFECT OF SELECTED THRIVE DIET FOODS

foods	highly alkaline-forming	alkaline-forming	neutral	slightly acid-forming
miscellaneous	Gingerroot	Apple cider vinegar	Herbs, dried (general)	
	Green tea	Balsamic vinegar	Miso paste	
		Garlic	Spice (general)	
	Herbs, fresh (general)			
	Rooibos			
	Yerba maté			

FOODS COMMON IN THE TYPICAL NORTH AMERICAN DIET

foods	slightly alkaline-forming	neutral	acid-forming	highly acid-forming
				Commercial breakfast cereals
				Pasta
				Refined wheat flour
grains				White rice
meat			Cold-water fish	Beef
			Venison	Pork
			Wild game	Poultry
				Shellfish
dairy			Milk, raw, unprocessed	Butter
				Cheese (all types)
				Cream
				Milk, pasteurized
sweeteners				Artificial sweeteners
				White sugar
miscellaneous			Synthetic multivitamins	Candy
				Coffee

FOODS COMMON IN THE TYPICAL NORTH AMERICAN DIET

foods	slightly alkaline-forming	neutral	acid-forming	highly acid-forming
				Margarine
				Peanuts (roasted)
				Prescription drugs
				Soft drinks
				Soy protein isolate
				Whey protein isolate

While I realize that most people who eat a typical North American diet do eat some alkalizing foods, such as fruit and vegetables, the amounts are rarely large enough to offset the acidity formed by the base of the diet. Even many so-called healthy diets, particularly those based heavily on cooked grains, keep the body in an overly acidic state, resulting is slowed cellular regeneration. Not all foods you eat need to be highly alkaline-forming; however, for optimal health, it is important that most of them are alkalizing.

As you can seen in the table on page 49, the acid-forming foods that are standard in the Thrive Diet register only as *slightly* acid-forming or less so. This is in opposition to the base ingredients of many common diets, which are usually highly acid-forming. Take pizza, for example. Compare the ingredients of a traditional pizza with the ones in a Thrive Diet pizza (the recipes begin on page 234). A conventional pizza is made from white flour, cheese, and processed meat—all cooked at a high temperature. These highly acid-forming ingredients combined with

Most modern diets are based on acid-forming foods, resulting in a stress response.

high-temperature cooking makes for a biologically taxing meal. A Thrive Diet pizza crust, on the other hand, is made from lentils and beets, and topped with fresh sun-dried tomato sauce and vegetables, then low-temperature baked.

proteins

As you will also notice in the table on page 49, alkaline-forming foods are foods that are in their most natural state—they have not been refined, chemically altered, or fortified. In contrast, many of the most acid-forming foods are manufactured and heavily processed. Protein-rich foods are made up of amino acids and are, as you might expect, more acid-forming. However, there are three questions you can ask in order to select the ones with the highest pH. First, has the food been processed? This is the greatest single determinant of its pH. If, for example, the food has had its fiber removed, thus raising its protein ratio, it will be more acid-forming. (The removal of nutrients has also, of course, made it less healthy.) The most common processing of a protein involves isolating it. This is done by removing the carbohydrate and fat, thereby creating protein isolates. Whey and soy protein powders are two types of protein isolates. You have likely seen these isolates in, ironically, health food stores. Popular with bodybuilders, isolates have been well marketed using the "more is better" rational. But it's not exactly rational. The isolation process involves high temperatures and usually chemicals. The resulting protein will have a significantly lower pH than it did before processing and will be acid-forming.

The second question to ask is, is the protein raw? Cooking protein can make it more acid-forming. Since pasteurization is a form of cooking, it is best to select unpasteurized sources. Raw is best, but if the protein needs to be pasteurized to kill bacteria, be sure that it is flash pasteurized only. Flash pasteurization is a process by which the protein is heated just long enough to reduce the proliferation of harmful bacteria—but not long enough to significantly affect protein quality. So, the first two questions consider the food's manufacturing. The less altered by processing and cooking, the better.

The third question is, does the protein source contain chlorophyll? Since chlorophyll is very alkalizing, a protein containing it will have a high pH. An easy way to determine chlorophyll content is to look at its color. Is it green? Hemp, many types of peas, legumes, dark green leafy vegetables, and seaweeds, although high in amino acids and therefore protein, are also high in chlorophyll, balancing the pH.

Natural proteins with a relatively high pH include sprouts (any kind—nuts, seeds, legumes); algae such as chlorella and spirulina; grasses such as wheat, oat, and barley; cooked legumes (though cooked legumes are not as alkaline-forming as sprouted legumes); flaxseeds and hemp. Hemp protein, for example, is not isolated and so remains in a relatively natural state, retaining its alkalinity. Also, hemp is raw, another factor contributing to its higher pH.

Daily consumption of protein with a relatively high pH (more alkaline) will minimize the body's acidity. A diet high in leafy green vegetables will also help ensure the system remains alkaline.

acid-forming foods and digestion

When acid-forming foods are consumed (starting with digestion and continuing through to elimination), they produce toxins that the body must deal with. Refined and processed foods are, as you know, highly acid-forming, and devoid of any usable nutrients, but they retain their caloric value. As well, denatured foods not only instantly *create* an acidic environment within the body because of their chemical composition, but they also *contain* toxins, leading to premature aging through cell degeneration. Most prescription drugs, artificial sweeteners, and synthetic vitamin and mineral supplements are also highly acid-forming.

As the body carries out normal functions such as movement and digestion, it naturally becomes increasingly acidic: Acid formation is a natural by-product of a healthy metabolism. This normal biological function becomes a problem only when an inordinate amount of food is consumed. As I mentioned earlier, nutrient-dense, high net-gain food is key. The lower the net gain of the food, the more that must be consumed to obtain all the nutrients the body needs. This leads not only to an overconsumption of empty calories but also to the digestion of more food than is necessary. The more food that passes through the system, the more acidic the body will become.

bone health

Balanced pH plays a major role in bone health. Studies indicate that it is not a lack of dietary calcium, as is commonly thought, but stress and overconsumption of acid-forming foods and supplements that lead to most cases of poor bone health and osteoporosis. The blood will always remain neutral—this is imperative for survival—so if the body is consistently fed acid-forming, denatured foods and supplements, or encounters stress from other sources, it must take measures to ensure a neutral blood pH is maintained. In doing so, the body pulls calcium, the mineral is our body that is most alkaline, from the bones. Over time, the bones weaken as a result of this survival mechanism.

The conventional way of treating low calcium levels and osteoporosis is to "take" more calcium, usually in the form of supplements. The calcium in tablets is usually derived from oyster shells, bovine bone meal, coral, or dolomite (a type of rock), all of which are extremely hard and unnatural for the body to assimilate—they are not food. The large size of these supplements and, with some types, the number recommended for daily intake is a testament to their poor bioavailability. The body must work very hard to get calcium from these sources.

pH levels and enjoyment of life

Diet has the greatest impact on the body's pH level; however, there are other contributing factors. Maintaining a positive attitude and setting time aside to do an activity you enjoy on a regular basis will promote pH balance within the body. Taking time out of a busy schedule to do something pleasurable yet seemingly unproductive is actually a key element in improved health and longevity—and therefore greater productivity. Of course, if you enjoy your busy schedule, it will be less stress-producing than if you perceive it as daunting—what might seem a foreboding schedule to someone else may be a source of pleasure for you. If you enjoy working through the night, then there is no need to rest. This further underscores the value of enjoying what you do for the long-term sake of your health.

> pH balance is a major factor in building and maintaining bone health.

Other ways of encouraging alkalinity within the body are—

- deep-breathing exercises,
- yoga,
- light stretching,
- meditation,
- any other activities you enjoy.

ratios of alkaline-forming to acid-forming foods

Some experts suggest that our diet consist of 75 percent alkaline-forming foods and 25 percent acid-forming foods. I believe that trying to hit a specific dietary ratio is unnecessary. This is partly because, as I noted above, several factors other than food affect the body's pH. Stress in general has a significant impact on pH. The body will sway to the acidic side even if the diet is alkaline-forming when it is confronted with high levels of non-nutritional stress. In this case, trying to hit a certain dietary ratio of alkaline-forming to acid-forming foods will not be useful. Simply adopting the Thrive Diet is the simplest thing you can do to ensure the body's pH is neutral or slightly alkaline.

one-step nutrition

One-step nutrition is the term I use to describe food containing nutrients already in a form usable by the body, with no breaking down required. The nutrients get into the body and go straight to work.

Nutrients in foods in a typical North American diet are in a form that the body must first break down and convert before it can utilize them.

form in typical north american food		**form the body uses directly, prevalent in the thrive diet**
Complex carbohydrates	must convert to ...	Simple carbohydrate
Fat	must convert to ...	Fatty acids
Protein	must convert to ...	Amino acids

By consuming one-step foods, the body is fueled and able to rebuild efficiently. Requiring minimal energy to become usable and assimilated, foods containing one-step nutrients in effect provide the body with *more* energy by helping conserve energy. Gaining the greatest amount of energy from the least amount of food is the goal of the Thrive Diet.

Food has three main components: carbohydrate, protein, and fat. Carbohydrate, accounting for most of the food we eat, consists of sugar, starch, and fiber. The ratio of each in any given food varies. Generally, fruits have high sugar levels; bread, pasta, and rice have large amounts of starch, also known as complex carbohydrate; and vegetables are fiber-rich.

The base of the Thrive Diet pyramid (see Chapter 1, page 40) consists of fibrous vegetables. In addition to fiber, these foods deliver a large amount of chlorophyll, vitamins, and minerals, as well as fluid to help maintain hydration. For fuel, though, fruit is the food of choice. This is in keeping with the Thrive Diet's one-step principle, since it is easily digestible and rich in simple carbohydrate. Also known as simple sugar, simple carbohydrate is a one-step nutrient; it can be directly used by the body for fuel. Conversely, the body must break down complex carbohydrate into simple carbohydrate before it can burn it, which takes extra work. Extra work requires energy, leaving the body with less.

Whole, unrefined complex carbohydrates do have their place in our diet, though. Pseudograins and other seeds, Thrive Diet staples, provide high-quality protein but also contain complex carbohydrate, yet in a form that is more easily used by the body than traditional sources, such as wheat. In addition, vitamins and minerals found in fruit and vegetables are nicely complemented by those present in unrefined whole grains such as brown rice, and in starchy vegetables such as sweet potatoes and yams. Therefore, these foods are found at the top of the Thrive Diet pyramid: They are part of the diet, but their role, in terms of quantity, is modest.

Foods Rich in Simple Carbohydrate

Bananas
Berries
Dates
Figs
Mangos
Papayas
Pineapples

Protein, which reconstructs body tissue, is the body's building nutrient. Regeneration is an ongoing process: In the course of the day, through normal wear and tear, body tissue is constantly being broken down and rebuilt. From the food we eat, the body converts protein into amino acids for use; it cannot utilize protein directly. We can help our body speed the regeneration process and be more efficient in the fabrication of new cells by eating foods rich in amino acid—one-step foods. This way, the body does not have to expend energy to convert protein into amino acids. Greens have the highest percentage of amino acids per ounce of any food. However, since greens do not weigh much, they need to be eaten daily to reap the full benefits that their amino acid profile offers. Eating a large green salad each day is part of the Thrive Diet.

Foods Rich in Amino Acids

Hemp

Leafy greens (all those composing the base of the Thrive Diet pyramid; see page 40)

Sprouts: legumes, pseudograins, seeds

Dietary fat is necessary for the lubrication of joints and for the activation of fat-soluble vitamins. It is also drawn on as an energy source when the body's carbohydrate supply is low. As with carbohydrate and protein, dietary fat must be broken down into a form the body can utilize. The body breaks fat into fatty acids—nutrients it can assimilate and put to work. Consuming fat sources that are directly made up of fatty acids is advantageous since the body will be able to make instant use of them.

Foods Rich in Fatty Acids

Seeds and oil:
- Flaxseed
- Hemp
- Pumpkin seed
- Sesame seed

The most complete, balanced form of one-step nutrition is sprouted foods. Raw, enzyme-rich sprouts are plentiful in all three food components: simple carbohydrate, amino acids, and fatty acids. They are predigested (as some describe it) so the body does not have to produce its own enzymes, plus the nutrients are in a usable form—a considerable net gain in total energy supplied by the food. (Contrast this to processed, cooked proteins that the body must break down before they can be utilized, creating a significant loss in energy efficacy.) Spouted legumes such as chickpeas, lentils, and mung beans are excellent. The sprouting process converts the complex carbohydrate in legumes into simple carbohydrate, the protein into usable amino acids, and the fat into fatty acids, requiring no extra work on the body's part and therefore raising the net gain. Foods rich in essential fatty acids, such as flaxseed, can be sprouted as well for a premium, usable fuel source. Indeed, essential fatty acids are a superior source of healthy energy.

nutrient-dense whole foods will keep you satisfied

"You are what you eat." This is true, but there's more to it than that. Eating food that is not efficiently absorbed and assimilated by the body will greatly limit its effectiveness. The way to ensure you are getting maximum return on your eating—the most energy out of your food—is simpler than you might think. In fact, the simpler the better. As a general rule, the less that has been done to your food, the better its return will be.

Food with low nutrient value is a major factor in escalating obesity rates. This serious health concern, though not desirable, does serve a purpose: It sends a clear message that something is out of balance. For optimum health and lasting benefits, the cause of the problem must be addressed, not the symptom. Specifically treating extra body fat, as many diets do, is treating only the symptom. Excess body fat is a clear indication that optimal health has not been achieved, and to treat it without creating a healthier lifestyle on a holistic level is merely spot-treating. Food cravings, usually for sugary or starchy foods, are often a telltale sign that the diet lacks nutrients or is tired. Cravings and chronic hunger, if not addressed, will lead to weight gain and fatigue in the short term and, in the long term, any number of health problems.

We are inundated with nutrient-lacking foods, most of them processed and refined foods eaten for convenience sake. We know that fresh fruit, vegetables, legumes, seeds, essential fatty acids, and compete protein are part of a healthy diet, but we believe we simply don't have time to prepare meals that reflect this. The result? A low-energy yet overfed society.

Nutrient-lacking convenience foods, ubiquitous in our society, cause us to lack energy.

Appetite will diminish as the quality of food improves. A real-life example of a stable of racehorses in the United States nicely illustrates this. These horses had impressive track records, and since the stakes in horse racing can be high, the horses were pushed hard in their daily training. But the trainers noticed an odd habit the horses had adopted. They had all, within the same week, started gnawing on the wood beams of their stables. Their trainers didn't know what to make of this peculiar behavior. They initially thought the horses needed more food. And so extra food was given to them, but the gnawing was relentless. By now, the horses were becoming overweight: They no longer looked like the racehorses they were but like draft horses.

After much deliberation, the trainers determined that the grain being fed to the horses had been grown in over-farmed soil and had been milled to the point of significant fiber loss. It therefore lacked essential nutrients. When a new source of nutrient-dense grain was found and this grain was fed to the horses, their appetites quickly dropped off and the gnawing stopped. The horses' chronic hunger had been due to lack of nutrition, not lack of food.

When supplied with many vitamins and minerals, the body will be properly fueled, and it will not require as much food. Its hunger mechanism will signal that it's no longer hungry. The Thrive Diet is built on a base of nutrient-dense foods. Simply by following the 12-Week Meal Plan, you will be well nourished, and fat loss will come naturally.

whole foods for complete nourishment

The healthiest way to meet nutritional needs is to simply eat a diet rich in whole foods. Food-sourced vitamins and minerals are superior to their laboratory-created counterparts. As I noted earlier, many calcium supplements are derived from nonfood sources—oyster shells, bovine bone meal, or dolomite—none of which the body is able to use efficiently. Again, the more work the body must do to assimilate nutrients, the less usable energy it will be left with. Salt is another illustration of this. Salt derived from the earth or the sea is often added to food during processing; salt is rarely consumed in its alternative form—plants. Yet, that is a much better way to get sodium in your diet: Let the plant draw and assimilate it and other minerals from the soil or sea, doing most of the work for you. My favorite source of sodium is raw dulse. A sea vegetable, dulse is exceptionally healthy, offering a plethora of minerals that help prolong hydration and therefore endurance.

"I just want to make completely sure that I'm getting all the vitamins I need, so I take every supplement available, the more the better. My body will just excrete what it doesn't use." I hear this often. And while this is true of water-soluble vitamins (vitamins B and C) and minerals such as potassium, chloride, and sodium, fat-soluble vitamins and certain minerals, such as iron, are not so readily excreted. Nevertheless, it is a common practice, especially for athletes. But at what cost?

While it's not a high-energy cost for a healthy body to flush out unneeded vitamins and minerals, it is still a cost. The body is under great stress to recover from workouts, rebuild cells, and keep the immune system strong, and the last thing it needs is another job. Most people take too many supplements in an effort to speed regeneration. Often they just interfere with that process, prolonging the time needed for complete recovery.

An excess of synthetic fat-soluble vitamins (A, D, E, and K) in the system can have a considerably more negative effect than those that are water-soluble. Unlike water-soluble vitamins, fat-soluble vitamins remain in the system for a long period—any surplus being stored in the body's fat cells, and possibly resulting in toxicity. General fatigue and a weakened immune system are the milder effects of such toxicity. Effects of more serious toxicity range from hemorrhaging to severe reduction in intestinal flora.

Toxicity resulting from an overconsumption of fat-soluble vitamins is next to impossible when whole foods are the source. Fiber prevents overeating: It's hard to eat a large amount of fiber-rich food since it swells in the stomach, filling it up.

Look through any sport or fitness magazine and you will undoubtedly notice advertisements making claims such as "improves performance by 20 percent." Even articles that may carry more credibility than advertisements make such claims. Do these vitamin and mineral supplements improve athletic performance? If a healthy diet is already being eaten, the answer is no.

Usually funded by manufacturers, many of the studies cited in these advertisements and articles were performed on people who had a deficiency in the particular vitamin or mineral being tested, making the test results somewhat misleading. And a person who has extremely low levels of any kind of essential nutrient will not perform to his or her full potential, whether in athletic competition or simply day-to-day living. Once the person gets the nutrient he is lacking, his symptoms will alleviate and he will experience better performance.

These claims—the gains made when the particular product is taken—are not false or even a bending of the truth. But they are results that are not typical for a healthy person who eats a sensible diet. By following the Thrive Diet, you won't need to take any supplements to enhance performance—the Thrive Diet supplies all the nutrients your body needs.

A whole-food diet will provide the body with all the nutrients it needs.

determining common food sensitivities

With symptoms ranging from a mild flu-like condition to headaches, difficulty sleeping, bloating, and fatigue, food sensitivities are becoming increasingly common in North America. Corn, wheat (and gluten, the protein found in wheat), dairy products, and soy have become so common in our food chain that many people have developed an intolerance to them through overconsumption. (Over time, however, the opposite might happen—we might build up a resistance to them.)

A standard practice in naturopathic medicine is to eliminate all sources of common allergens from the diet. This is a logical way to determine if the patient has an allergy or sensitivity to commonly eaten foods. Sensitivity can be defined as an unpleasant reaction caused by eating food that the body does not have the specific enzymes or chemicals to digest properly. Unlike an allergic reaction, a sensitivity does not affect the immune system. Food allergies are not usually a major problem because they often become evident immediately upon consuming the food: There's no mistaking them, the symptoms—tingling in the mouth, swelling of the tongue and throat, difficulty breathing, abdominal cramps, vomiting—come on quickly. Stop consuming the problem food and the problem is solved. The symptoms of a specific food sensitivity, however, might not become evident for a few days or a week after consumption, making its source difficult to trace. Food sensitivities, therefore, can be extremely difficult to immediately identify and eliminate, and in these cases, the strategy of eliminating common allergens from the diet is useful.

For a few years, I had what I thought to be a bad case of hay fever each spring. I didn't really think too much of it. Then came the year I learned about food sensitivities, and I eliminated all common allergens from my diet. That year, spring arrived, but my hay fever did not. As it turned out, the congestion I had experienced in previous years was from a sensitivity to corn and not because of rising pollen counts. In spring I typically cycle more—and, before my food-elimination experiment, I drank a lot of a so-called endurance-enhancing sport drink. The first ingredient of this drink was maltodextrin, a cheap sugar derivative made from corn and, as I found out, the precipitator of my hay fever–like symptoms.

Many people have a food sensitivity but don't know it. "Not feeling quite up to par" is often how they describe the way they feel. They rule out diet as being the culprit since it has remained constant—unchanged—for a number of years. Some people blame environmental factors such as dust or pollen. The dull symptoms, or sometimes simply a state of malaise, can persist for years; since they just make certain activities a bit more difficult without actually preventing them, no action is taken. But it is precisely the unchanging diet that is behind the symptoms.

If you think you may have a food sensitivity, try eliminating common allergens—corn, wheat/gluten, dairy products, soy, active yeast, and peanuts—from your diet for 10 days or so. Have a look at the ingredients of the manufactured foods you are consuming; you are likely consuming one or more of these irritants at every meal. The Thrive Diet recipes are free of these allergens; the 12-Week Meal Plan on page 167 will point you in the right direction.

Why are some foods likely to cause sensitivities? In short, because they are no longer in their natural state or are being eaten by someone other than the intended consumer.

corn

Corn, or maize, in its current state is, believe it or not, a man-made food. Native Americans in central Mexico crossed grasses to produce a crop that was better able to feed them. Early cobs were only an inch or two long and so produced little food, but over the course of about 7000 years, maize was cultivated to produce a larger cob and therefore a greater yield. This relatively new addition to the human diet causes an allergic reaction in some people.

High-fructose corn syrup, one of the most health-damaging derivatives of corn, is frequently used in sport drinks and other processed foods requiring a cheap sweetener. Corn derivatives are used in upward of 90 percent of processed food, and people who eat a standard diet often develop an intolerance and sensitivity to it. However, if your body accepts corn with no adverse reaction, there is no need to avoid healthful whole corn, such as fresh corn on the cob.

wheat and gluten

Gluten, the protein found in wheat, is difficult for some people to digest. High levels of gluten are not historically natural to our diet; they are a modern creation. Ancient grains such as spelt and barley contain small amounts of gluten, which most people can tolerate without any problem. Ancient grains can be a healthy addition to your diet if your system can tolerate small amounts of gluten. Wheat, however, is not a natural food. It has been "encouraged" to grow the way it does today to produce a better crop yield. As with corn, ancient grains were cultivated thousands of years ago to produce more food on less land, and the accompanying result was higher levels of gluten in the crop. Unfortunately, the consequence of eating it is often mild to severe digestive problems—ranging from simply feeling subpar to allergic reactions and celiac disease. Gluten-rich foods are also fairly acid-forming. Wheat, or a derivative, is in nearly all processed food.

dairy

Cow's milk comes from a lactating cow. Natural unpasteurized milk from a mother cow is an ideal source of nourishment—for the calf. When the milk is fed to humans, it is no longer being used as it was intended. Many people, especially adults, experience digestive problems when consuming cow's milk. The same holds true for goat's and sheep's milk, and products made from all these milks. It is common for people to have a food sensitivity because their body is not used to a certain food. Asians are most prone to dairy sensitivities since consuming dairy products has traditionally not been part of their culture: Their bodies have not had as much time to build up a resistance to it. Most people, of Asian origin or not, who eliminate dairy products find that they feel better and lose weight more easily. Most healthy bodies are capable of building a resistance to small amounts of dairy; however, in doing so it uses energy and reduces the effectiveness of the immune system.

soy

Soy has traditionally been eaten in Asia as a condiment, not as a main course. Since the Western world has embraced soy as a meat substitute, it has found its way into our diets on a large scale—as the base for imitation meat products, soy has become a staple for many who have made the shift from meat. I certainly view this as progress; however, some people have not experienced the vitality they were seeking when switching to a plant-based diet. Many North Americans who consumed soy at every meal developed a sensitivity to it over the course of a few years. Soy milk on cereal in the morning, a tofu burger for lunch, and a tofu stir-fry for dinner—these are common in the diet of newly health-conscious people.

Some experts are calling soy the new gluten, meaning that it is being used as filler in many processed foods. Even when not apparent, soy, as with gluten and corn, is in nearly all processed foods, and we risk developing an intolerance to it. However, eating organic tofu once a week or so as your only source of soy is a perfectly healthy option, if you don't have a sensitivity to it. I suggest you follow the Asian lead and have soy products as condiments to meals, not as the main course.

active yeast

There are two categories of yeast: inactive and active. Nutritional yeast is inactive, meaning that it is no longer growing. It is yeast that has been grown on molasses and then harvested and pasteurized, rendering it inactive. It will not feed on sugars in the body or promote *candida albicans*, a yeast-like fungus that lives in the digestive tract. It is a nutrient-packed healthy food (I discuss it in detail in Chapter 5, page 158).

Active yeast, on the other hand, is living and needs sugar to survive once in contact with moisture. Used to make bread dough rise, it is a standard ingredient in most baked goods. The yeast feeds on the sugar used when making bread, and it is not destroyed by the heat of baking; it enters our body when we eat the bread and survives by feeding on our body's sugars. This can cause yeast infections and candidiasis. Some people develop bloating and mild flu-like symptoms when they eat active yeast. However, if you do not experience any trouble from eating food containing active yeast, there is no reason to specifically eliminate it from your diet. If you do choose to eat baked goods containing yeast, be sure to eat those that are made from whole sprouted grains.

Standard diets can precipitate sensitivities caused by altered foods.

peanuts

Although still relatively low numbers of people are affected, peanut allergies and sensitivities are on the rise in North America, affecting children the most severely (though about 20 percent outgrow their allergy or sensitivity). Reactions from peanuts range from mild to severe—some people are affected by simply the presence of peanut-containing foods in the same room, thanks to air-borne peanut particles. The reason for such a severe reaction to peanuts is still not well understood. The immune systems of those people affected seem to perceive the peanut protein as a form of poison, an invader to the body. In response to the perceived threat, the body produces antibodies. When there is no real poison to fight, yet antibodies have been released, an allergic reaction is typical. Symptoms of the allergy include swelling around the eyes, difficulty breathing, and rash. Those who have a severe peanut allergy may experience restricted breathing, possibly even anaphylactic shock. For those of you who like peanut butter but have a peanut allergy, the Thrive Diet's Sunflower Seed Pâté is a good alternative (recipe on page 264).

It is estimated that upward of 98 percent of all processed foods in the typical North American diet contains at least one common allergen. In fact, corn and wheat by-products can be found in all conventional fast food. The Thrive Diet is not based on any of these foods. A few of the recipes contain oats, which do contain gluten, but I also suggest substitutions.

eliminating biological debt

I use the term *biological debt* to refer to a state that the body goes into after energy from stimulation has dissipated. Often brought about by eating refined sugar or drinking coffee to gain energy in the short term, biological debt is a state of fatigue. Unfortunately, it is a state that many North Americans are accustomed to living in.

For long-term health and vitality, we need to understand the difference between two types of energy: one obtained from stimulation, the other from nourishment. As a general rule, the more processed the food is, the more stimulating its effect will be on the nervous system, and the less nourishing. In contrast, the more natural and whole a food is—raw and sprouted being the best—the less stimulating and the more nourishing it will be. Because of our insatiable desire for quick, convenient energy "on the go," our streets are crammed with coffee, donut, and fast food establishments. This solves the convenience problem and offers a short-term energy solution through stimulation. However, it does nothing to help with the payment inevitably required by the body if this route is taken regularly. The body can subsist on stimulating, nutrient-absent food only so long before becoming either exhausted or sick—and where the body goes, the mind is sure to follow.

In the afternoon, about 3 P.M., lunch has started to wear off, and hunger and fatigue is creeping in. Reaching for either a cup of coffee, a snack high in refined carbohydrates, or both is common. Coffee and refined carbohydrates give a short energy boost but stress the body. Coffee also raises cortisol levels, which lowers the immune system, making the body more vulnerable to infection and eventually leading to the storage of body fat. Refined carbohydrates cause an insulin spike that will elevate cortisol levels. Excessive consumption of coffee and refined carbohydrates will also result in inflammation, a key cause of premature aging (see page 46).

Many of us are in a constant state of biological debt. Simply put, it is a huge contributing factor to overall stress and therefore has become a major precipitator of fatigue, weight gain, and compromised health in general. If untreated, it can lead to serious diseases.

One measure of health is having cost-free energy—energy that lasts and does not have to be "stoked" continually with processed carbohydrates, manufactured sugar, or caffeine. The stoking of energy can end in one result only: less energy. Ironically, many so-called energy foods are the biggest energy-suckers. The high level of processing they undergo ensures that their shelf life is dramatically extended, but this is accompanied by a marked decline in nutritional quality. These foods are certainly not part of a sustainable, high-energy diet.

While convenient, many energy bars offer nothing more nutritional than what candy bars offer. High in calories supplied from adrenal-fatiguing refined sources, most energy bars provide energy for the short term (anything with calories will) but, after a person consumes them for several months, will bring about fatigue. The processing they go through in manufacturing, which lowers their pH and destroys their enzymes, make them a strain on both the immune and digestive

Stress Triggers and Cortisol Levels

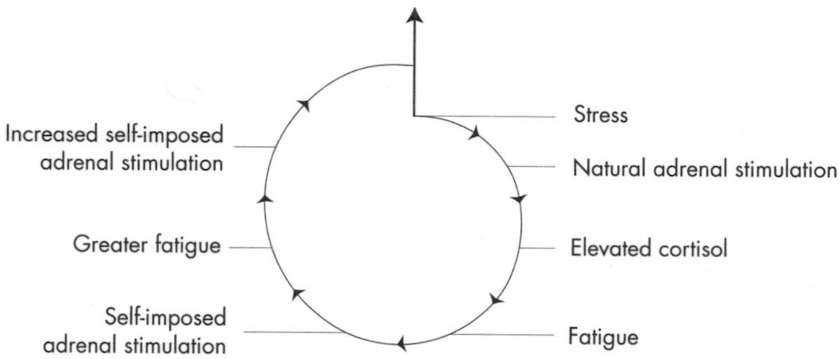

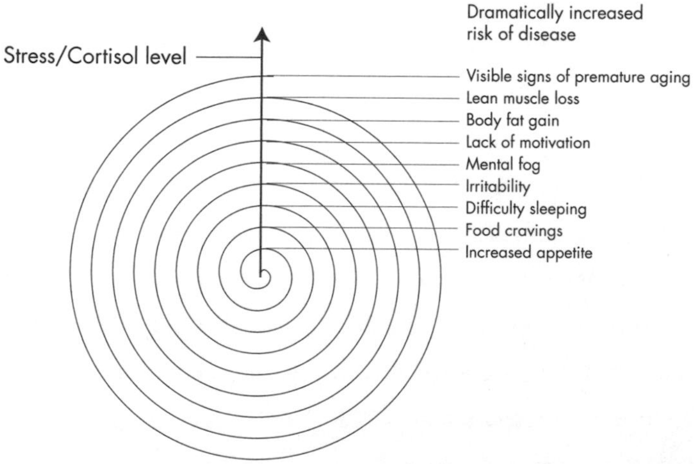

systems, rendering them a low net-gain, stressful food. Superior energy-maximizing foods are those that offer sustainable energy, not quick bouts of stimulation. High net-gain whole foods provide a platform on which to build long-term sustainable vitality. In the recipe section of this book, you will find several recipes for high net-gain energy bars, ones that I've made for myself for several years.

As you can see from the top illustration on page 72, stress triggers the spiral. As you read in Chapter 1, for the average North American, 40 percent of that stress can be directly linked to diet. With the first onset of stress comes natural adrenal stimulation, which is not unhealthy in small doses. The rise in cortisol level, however, always results in fatigue. That is, any kind of stimulation, regardless of how dramatic or mild, produces short-term energy, but it is *always* followed by fatigue. The degree of fatigue depends on the degree of stimulation: The greater the stimulation, the greater the fatigue. The healthiest things a person can do at this point is rest and remove the elements causing the stress, such as poor diet. Yet, this is when most people turn to self-imposed adrenal stimulants such as coffee and refined foods, to regain energy. This leads to greater fatigue and then more stimulation. The circle is complete.

Stress leads to fatigue, which leads to self-imposed stimulation. From there the spiral begins and the symptoms' negative effects compound.

Each time the circle completes itself, the severity of the condition rises, creating an incremental decline in health and an increased risk factor for serious disease. As the bottom illustration on page 72 shows, the first completion of the circle will likely result only in a slightly increased appetite. The next time round will result in cravings, likely for starchy, refined foods. Sequential passes involve difficulty sleeping, irritability, mental fog, lack of motivation, body fat gain, lean muscle loss, visible signs of premature aging, and sickness. Each round produces a more severe symptom, on top of the previous ones, compounding the effect. If this cycle of chronically elevated cortisol levels is allowed to continue, tissue degeneration, depression, chronic fatigue syndrome, and even diseases such as cancer can develop.

The Thrive Diet is about breaking this cycle by providing energy through nourishment, without artificial stimulation. This, along with simply being properly rested by getting efficient sleep (because of a reduction in stress through better diet), will prevent a spiral such as this from developing.

You have undoubtedly experienced stimulation of the sort I'm talking about here. Unexpectedly hearing a loud noise, for example, when the room is quiet, you might feel a sudden rush of energy. This is left over from our primal survival mechanism. Your body assumes the loud noise is a threat and so prepares you for action by engaging the adrenal glands to draw more energy. Even listening to loud music is stimulation. Listening to heavy music immediately before an event *will* better prepare an athlete. Heavy music played at high volume is perceived as a threat by the body and gets the adrenaline pumping, readying the athlete for competition. In the short term, stress will reduce the effectiveness of the pain receptors; this is advantageous to athletes, and the benefit of being biologically scared. However, if the heavy music is played too far in advance of a race or other athletic event, even the day before, it will tire the athlete before the competition begins.

Many types of classical music played at a low volume have been shown to have a positive physical effect on the body. Several studies have shown the effectiveness of music therapy in helping reduce stress-related symptoms and boost relaxation.

A SEEMINGLY MUNDANE ACTIVITY, watching TV, has been receiving a lot of interest over the past few years. Many health professionals believe children in North America watch too much TV and that this is linked to childhood obesity. This makes sense: Children who come home from school and sit on the couch in front of the TV, rather than playing soccer, for example, are simply not as physically active. To make matters worse, most children snack when they watch TV. But many studies on the TV-watching habits of children stopped there: The sedentary nature of TV viewing was determined to be the culprit for kids' weight gain. However, I believe the TV itself is largely to blame. Watching TV is stimulating, especially if it's a violent program.

As you have read, one of the first signs of stress is greater energy, closely followed by fatigue. And when children become tired, what are they likely to do? Usually, they will eat something sugary for an energy boost. By doing this, they further stimulate and in turn tire the adrenals, resulting in greater fatigue. Simply put, they are overstressed by being undernourished and overstimulated.

Violent video games have gained immense popularity in the past decade or two. Is this because children are becoming more naturally violent? Or is simply because they're tired, and subconsciously drawn to the "energy" supplied by stimulation? The best way to help children out of the vicious circle created is providing them with proper nutrition. Because of the unstimulating nature of most healthy foods, overstimulated children will likely resist them at first. But once they grow accustomed to their new diet—as with adults, only magnified—the subconscious desire to harness energy by stimulating the adrenals will diminish.

All the recipes in this book are healthy for children; some are especially kid-friendly:

- Banana Chocolate Pancakes (recipe, page 213)—these are packed with sustainable nutrition to start the day off right.
- Energy Pudding and Recovery Pudding (recipes in Chapter 5, pages 125 and 126)—a tasty nutrient-packed snack, these puddings are easy to pack as part of a school lunch. For children, I recommend the non–yerba maté version.
- Apple Cinnamon and Banana Bread energy bars (recipes, pages 228 and 229)—these bars are high-quality portable nutrition, perfect for school snacks and lunches.
- Chocolate Almond and Tropical Pineapple Mango smoothies (recipes, pages 222 and 223)—these are great for breakfast, after school, or after sports practice.

The less stimulation a person has in everyday life, the greater impact stimuli will have on the body. This is good. It means the person is living a low-stress life, and we know the benefits of that. But there's more to it. It also means that considerably less stimulation is needed to evoke a stress response from the adrenal glands. One of the body's most resourceful traits is its ability to adapt. Acclimatizing to stimulation is no exception.

Here's an example. When you turn on a light in a dark room, it seems very bright, although it really is no brighter than usual. Similarly, when ambient sound levels are low, the body's sense of hearing is heightened. Have you ever noticed that sometimes the phone's ring sounds very loud, and at other times it sounds relatively quiet? The key word is *relatively*. Our body has the ability to adjust to much of what goes on around it. That our system automatically adapts to external stimuli serves us well; but if the adjustment is not in keeping with the stimuli, it can be to our detriment.

To calibrate its sensory system, the body must decide at what level it will sense stimuli. The only gauge the body has is through the information we feed it: sound, sight, touch, smell, and taste. Its decision is based on the level at which we supply that information. If we drink a daily cup of coffee to increase our energy, it won't take long before its effect is diminished—before one cup of coffee will no longer serve the jolt it once did. It might seem logical, then, to drink a second cup to get the "energy" that a single cup used to delivered. But where does this cycle end?

Our bodies are chronically overstimulated, yet most of us don't realize it—our bodies have adapted, but at a cost. Constantly having to climb to a new level to remain in the same place is a tough way to live, yet all too common. The way to fix this problem, to remove considerable stress from the body and in doing so increase energy, is to recalibrate the body.

The Thrive Diet is a recalibration diet. It is naturally non-stimulating so your body will re-establish its sensory system, functioning at a healthier, more energetic level—without the cell-damaging need for stimulation. Recalibration can be achieved by removing as many stimuli as possible for a set period. The obvious stimuli are caffeine and refined carbohydrate, but there are others. Using your current health as a guide, you can determine where you want to begin. Your current diet and stress level will determine how long recalibration will take. If you are a regular coffee drinker and refined-food eater, it will take longer than if you consume minimal amounts of coffee and processed foods. That's okay. Start slow and ease into it. Cleansing and withdrawal symptoms are common. If they are too intense, simply slow that rate at which you adopt the Thrive Diet. At the end of this chapter, I explain how to make the transition successfully.

The bottom line: Once the body's stress is reduced and stimulation is minimal, it will have a greater level of sustainable energy.

hydration

Hydration is an extremely important part of the regeneration process and therefore the Thrive Diet. When the body is properly hydrated, the blood is at the proper consistency, enabling its efficient distribution throughout the body. The cells of a hydrated body swell, causing an anabolic response (growth of muscle tissue), speeding up cellular renewal. As well, hydrated cells remain alkaline. A catabolic response (breakdown of muscle tissue) will occur if the cells become dehydrated, advancing degeneration. Maintaining blood volume through proper hydration also allows:

- red blood cells to deliver oxygen to muscles efficiently,
- delivery of nutrients throughout the body,
- removal of waste products such as carbon dioxide,
- proper hormone distribution.

With the Thrive Diet, in addition to water and water-dense foods, healthy blender drinks provide necessary fluid. The Thrive Diet 12-Week Meal Plan includes a smoothie each day. Smoothies are great for sipping throughout the morning or afternoon. As well as getting a break from water, you'll be supplying your body with easily digestible health-promoting nutrition.

While maintaining hydration is important, it's not necessary to drink large amounts of fluid. On the Thrive Diet, you will notice that thirst doesn't develop as often and isn't as intense when eating. This is because the diet is based on raw and whole foods, which retain much of their moisture content. For instance, fruit and vegetables, a predominant part of the diet, are filled with water. When food is cooked, especially at high temperature, it loses moisture and can even act as a sponge once consumed to pull water from the system, increasing your thirst. The removal of the hull and the germ in the processing of grains also removes moisture; when you consume processed grains, your body's need for fluids to aid in digestion increases. Many denatured foods are full of thirst-inciting sodium and chemical-derived additives such as MSG. Often added to enhance the flavor of near flavorless food (the flavor having been lost during the refining process), sodium is commonly used in excess.

Maintaining hydration is paramount, but *how* hydration is maintained is just as important. Drinks containing caffeine are diuretic and actually dehydrate the body. Alcohol is also a diuretic. You will need to drink more water than usual after drinking caffeinated or alcoholic beverages to replenish the fluid your body has lost. A diet rich in processed, high-temperature-cooked food requires the consumption of several quarts of fluid a day to overcome the lack of fluid in the diet and control thirst. But drinking large amounts of water or other fluids to compensate for the lack of moisture in food is hard on the digestive system. Fluid drunk during or immediately after eating will adversely affect the body's digestive efficacy, making the system work harder to do its job.

As I mentioned earlier, those who eat a "dry" diet, one in which the food contains almost no moisture, will likely find they are almost always thirsty, because their body requires more fluid. Many people find plain water boring, and this is when excess calories are often introduced into the diet, in the form of sugary fluids such as sodas and juices with sugar added.

So, does everyone need to drink eight glasses of water a day? I don't believe you should drink water if you are not thirsty. By eating a natural, whole-food diet, the body's fluid requirements will be taken care of.

lifestyle tips to complement the thrive diet

don't jeopardize health in its pursuit

Be cognizant of the cost of health. If you are on a rigid and inhibiting program, are the benefits worth it? Carrying and having to remember to take numerous pills several times a day, or sticking to your exercise program regardless of all that unfolds in your life—is that healthy? Often we force ourselves to follow a regime even if we don't like it. Yet ironically, in its pursuit, health—and therefore performance—is compromised. If all else is equal, happy people are healthier people than unhappy people. Even the ideal exercise and diet program will not be beneficial if it's not enjoyable.

exposure to natural light

Exposure to natural light is essential for optimal health. Some experts consider sunlight a nutrient, as vital for well-being as certain dietary nutrients. Sunlight, when it enters our eyes, prompts our endocrine system to produce hormones that help regulate basic body function and maintain a healthy immune system.

Vitamin D, also known as the sunshine vitamin, is synthesized in our bodies when our skin is exposed to ultraviolet light. An essential component for calcium absorption and utilization, vitamin D is found in certain foods, but it is best obtained from sunlight.

People who have limited exposure to natural light—a common thing, given the prevalence of unnatural lighting indoors—often notice a decline in their mood. Natural light instigates the production of serotonin in the body, the hormone that, when released into our bloodstream, makes us feel good. As discussed in Chapter 1, once serotonin production drops, depression, weight gain (through increased appetite), and cluttered thought patterns are common. Also, as with the absence of any nutrient essential for health, the lack of natural light will eventually induce a stress response.

I try to make sure my skin gets adequate exposure to sunlight. This is easy when my training volume is high. But in the off-season, which is the wintertime where I live, I notice my energy declines unless I spend time in full-spectrum light. As with many things, however, some is good but more is not necessarily better. Exposing your skin to sunlight for about 10 minutes, two to three times a week, will provide your body with the sunlight it needs. Even on cloudy days, the sun's rays have a positive effect on exposed skin. But be sure not to overexpose your skin to direct sun; the resulting sunburn will result in the creation of free radicals in the body. And as the earth's ozone layer continues to deplete, the rate at which our skin will burn will increase.

darkness for improved sleep and recovery

Melatonin is a hormone produced in the pineal gland, a small endocrine gland in the brain. Its release is dependent on the amount of light the body is exposed to. As light fades toward the end of the day, melatonin is released. This melatonin helps prepare the body for sleep by reducing alertness and slightly lowering body temperature. I find that my ability to get a good night's sleep is closely tied to the natural production of melatonin in my body. For this reason, I limit my exposure to light for at least an hour before bedtime.

Darkness releases melatonin, a powerful sleep-enhancing hormone and antioxidant.

For those of you who have trouble sleeping despite a nutrient-rich diet and stress-curtailing strategies, I recommend deep relaxation. About an hour before bedtime, dim the lights, keeping them just bright enough so that you can walk without bumping into anything. This dimming of the lights will trigger the release of melatonin in your body, which will help clear your mind of linear thought—the day's events will start to blur if you think about them. Sit comfortably, wherever you like, with eyes closed, then breathe with slow, controlled, full breaths and let your mind wander. If melatonin is doing its job, structured thought will be difficult. I generally practice deep relaxation for about 20 minutes, then go to bed and slip into a deep sleep. Meditating before bed will also help you relax.

Melatonin is a potent antioxidant. Harnessing its power not only evokes a deep, regenerating sleep, it also speeds recovery at the cellular level.

avoid too many changes at once

Stress breaks down the body to varying degrees. This is fine: It's how we grow stronger—at least, once we recover from it. Provided that you have the resources and know-how to facilitate recovery, this process is healthy. If you don't, it can be detrimental.

The computer makes for a good analogy. If a computer tries to download material from several websites at once, the delivery of all information is slowed. Similarly, the body can deal with only so many demands placed on it. To overwhelm it is to slow the delivery of all results. Unlike a computer though, the body is able to prioritize. If you have a viral infection such as the flu while you are weight training, the time your body needs to recover from the workout will be considerably longer than usual. This is because the body perceives the viral infection as more threatening to the body as a whole than the acute damage of muscle tissue caused by exercise. But since the body must repair the muscle tissue to at least some degree, the flu will linger slightly longer.

It is not in our best interest to take on projects that ultimately slow our progress. I use this premise when designing my training program: I work on one aspect, become proficient at it, and then move on to the next. A parallel can be drawn between the phasing approach to training and everyday life: If you are going through a stressful time at work, are just recovering from the flu, and have recently moved to a new city, it's not a good time to start training for a triathlon.

mind-body connection

Most days, someone is vying for our attention. From television commercials to pop-up internet advertisements to billboards, our senses are in high demand. Everywhere we look, someone is marketing something. But once we are conscious of a particular product, how much influence does marketing have on our perception of it? Apparently, a significant amount: The better the advertising campaign, the better the product is perceived to work.

The placebo effect is a good illustration of this. Numerous studies show that placebos have about a 30 percent success rate. This means that if 10 people have a headache and are each given a pill they are told will cure it, 3 of those people will feel better. The pill might be nothing more than a sugar pill, with no headache-curing properties; it is simply the person's belief that the pill will cure the headache that cures the headache. When well-thought-out marketing comes into play, the "placebo effect" will be higher—as high as 60 percent. Using impressive, scientific-sounding words and routinely making unsubstantiated claims, sport nutrition companies are among the most exploitive of this knowledge. But it works, and not just to sell their products, but in their products' application. Athletes who believe that they have more energy after taking a pill often do. Those who believe they can lift more weight sometimes can. Even more impressive, the *color* of the pill can play a role in the outcome: The color red is thought of as an "energy" pill, while blue pills have a calming effect, facilitating speedy recovery.

The opposite is also true: The body has a compelling effect on the mind. If the body is being stressed beyond a point from which it can reasonably recover, thinking will be altered. Brain chemistry, affecting mood and general outlook, becomes distorted when the body is stressed. I've certainly noticed this effect after weeks of high-volume training. My ability to think clearly and to reason, and my cognitive aptitude in general, becomes impaired.

Simply being aware of the mind-body relationship is helpful. Knowing that this relationship is as close as it is will shed light on why we sometimes think what we think, even if it is not always rational.

The mind can significantly influence physical perception. Reducing physical stress improves mental clarity.

healthy food makes a difference

Many people subscribe to the "If it's not broken, don't fix it" philosophy. This way of thinking does make sense in certain situations. However, it's not a sound approach when applied to something with a cumulative effect, like diet and nutrition; poor diet is in part responsible for many ailments. Yet, many people believe that if their heart is still beating, their diet must be okay. To a point this is true, but I think that most people would like more from life than just survival. We know that ambition and mood can be adversely affected by poor diet. Lack of motivation, and the belief that you can't change or that what you want to achieve is out of reach, is often nothing more than a sign of a chronically poor diet. How do you break the cycle? The answer is applied knowledge.

I know people who started eating "health food" a few days before a race, shocked their body with the sudden change, had a bad race, and then surmised, "Health food doesn't make a difference." Healthy food is not a drug. Even though the change it brings about is positive, it takes the body time to adapt. Be patient. Convert gradually to a healthy, whole food–based diet. Allow your body time to adjust. Your overall health can only improve. And over time, improved health will lead to improved performance.

It's true that some great athletes eat junk food. "Look at his diet, it's full of refined, processed foods and doesn't seem to hurt him," some people like to point out. I believe that these are cases of an athlete being great in spite of a poor diet, not because of it. Take cigarette smoking, for instance. I could start smoking today and I could probably smoke for years, possibly decades, before any clear-cut, directly related problems arose. There would be underlying health issues, but they may not appear to be symptoms of smoking. It would be wrong for me to conclude that because I smoke and seem okay, smoking is not unhealthy. Similarly with poor nutrition: Suboptimal performance will be the result in the short term, while the serious health problems will manifest later.

As you could probably guess, I'm an advocate of preventative methods. By eating nutrient-dense whole foods now, we continue to reduce chances of disease later in life and we extend our life expectancy.

applying the thrive diet

change is stress

The body perceives any physical deviation from the routine as stress. Even if the change is a positive one, the body must adapt. The best way for someone who has smoked for many years to quit, for example, is to gradually reduce the amount of nicotine in her system. This is what the nicotine patch does—it slowly weans the person off cigarettes' addictive properties. With this method, the chances of success are greatly improved, simply because withdrawal stress is reduced.

A cold-turkey approach to quitting smoking is often not successful and can possibly be counterproductive. That it is easier and less stressful (and therefore healthier) to continue to smoke seems illogical. Yet, the smoker who instantly quits will experience more stress than the one who quits gradually by continuing to smoke but at a reduced rate. Over time, the body will adapt to the stress of withdrawal, overcome it, and be healthier. The point is, it takes time.

The same goes for nutrition. When you adopt a new way of eating, it takes time for your body to adapt. If you're following the Thrive Diet, the body will also need to contend with detoxification. Detoxification is the body's elimination of the toxins accumulated over years of consuming poor-quality food. It is a tremendously positive process. Our body is equipped with coping mechanisms that allow it to function as optimally as it can, given the nourishment it gets. The first few days of an optimal diet may not be pleasant. Years of eating less than ideal foods have rendered our body nutritionally stressed. The poorer the quality of your previous diet, the longer the detoxification process. It will likely take people converting from a typical North American diet to an exclusively whole-food plant-based diet more than six weeks to cleanse their body of toxins.

Chlorophyll in particular has a cleansing effect, helping the body extract toxins from the liver. As toxins are removed, withdrawal symptoms will be intensified, but overall withdrawl will be shorter. Eating chlorophyll-rich foods have been shown to help people break the addiction to nicotine and stop smoking.

Common detoxification symptoms include headache, bloating, diarrhea, nausea, fatigue, and sleep disturbances. It's important to remember that detoxification involves cleansing symptoms. Severe symptoms, however, are an indication that you should reduce the rate at which you are implementing the change. Keep in mind, though, that the worse you feel initially, the more there is to be gained.

adapting to the thrive diet

When first starting on the Thrive Diet, don't eliminate any specific food; rather, simply add Thrive Diet foods. Over time, the body will begin to crave high net-gain foods and lose interest in processed foods. Also, by making high net-gain foods a large part of the diet, there will simply be no room for others. The body will get all the nutrition it needs from the new diet and then turn off its hunger mechanism. At this point, eating more is unnecessary and even undesirable. But until the body breaks its habit of eating for reasons other than nourishment, such as tiredness or elevated stress, lingering cravings are normal. Once the body becomes better nourished on the Thrive Diet, these cravings will fade, as their underlying cause—stress and fatigue—will have been greatly reduced.

If your current diet already includes several elements of the Thrive Diet, you can begin by following the program closely. If, however, the way you are eating is in glaring contrast to the Thrive Diet, start by incorporating a few elements at a time. For instance, you might start with a nutrient-rich smoothie each day in place of a meal or a less-healthy snack, gradually incorporating more green foods into your diet, including having a salad a day. This allows your body and your mind to adapt slowly to the change. As you progress and feel comfortable, continue trying new ingredients and adding more Thrive Diet elements to your routine. Before you know it, you will be on the program and reaping the rewards.

recalibration: ease into it

The Thrive Diet involves recalibration—removing stimuli, including caffeine and refined carbohydrate. Since the body is used to being stimulated by food, it will likely feel more tired than usual for the first few days of recalibration, perhaps even irritated. This is normal. It is best not to recalibrate when other stressors in your life are high. Wait for a calm period.

A few summers ago, even though my diet was good, I recalibrated it to a further level, just as an experiment. For three days I ate nothing containing sugar—not even fruit. The result was a calm and productive state. At the end of the three days, I ate a few blueberries. Taking in just a small amount of sugar in the form of fruit had an immediate stimulating effect. It was like what I used to experience when I drank a cup of coffee. I'm not suggesting cutting back on fruit. But this experiment does nicely underscore the value of recalibration.

> Eliminating stimulating foods from our diets will provide a platform on which the Thrive Diet will be most successful.

Reducing stimuli so that our body becomes more sensitive to it translates into easily obtainable energy through natural foods. That the body's perception of the input has changed is key: *You* decide how you want your body to respond to various inputs. Food, of course, is one of the largest inputs. By recalibrating, we control its effect on our body and mind.

getting started on the thrive diet

general guidelines

Keep these general guidelines in mind as you embark on the Thrive Diet:

- Consume enough nutrients to support your activity level and the biological regeneration of your cells, to reduce biological age.
- Meet nutritional needs by consuming nutrient-dense whole foods, rather than supplementing with tablets.
- Avoid denatured foods—refined, processed foods.
- Gain energy through nourishment, not stimulation.
- Eat efficient foods: Increase energy by conserving it in digestion and assimilation.
- Recalibrate by reducing your intake of sugary and starchy foods.

specific guidelines

The specific guidelines below will help you plan your daily diet:

Eat throughout the day. By eating several small meals each day, as well as snacks, you will never be too full or get too hunger. Frequent eating helps maintain energy levels and will result in a smaller amount of food being consumed than if you were to eat three full meals a day. This is also a good way to ease digestive strain and spread nutrients throughout the day, improving their absorption rate.

Use the 12-Week Meal Plan as a guide. All the recipes in this book will help get you started on the Thrive Diet. Several recipes include variations, and don't be afraid to experiment further. If you follow the general guidelines above, and the Thrive Diet's guiding principles, listed on page 40, there is no end to the nutritious and tasty meals you can create.

Drink a nutritious smoothie each day. A daily nutrient-rich smoothie will ensure the body gets all the nourishment it needs in a whole-food form. The smoothies suggested in this book are not meant as a supplement to whole food: They *are* whole foods, just blended. Daily nourishment in the form of liquid will help take the strain off your digestive system, thereby providing even greater energy.

Eat a big green salad each day. Packed with chlorophyll, a leafy, green salad is among the healthiest of foods. Eating a big salad a day will boost overall health. It will help build new blood cells and keep the regeneration process going. High in fiber and minerals, salads are part of the base of the Thrive Diet pyramid (see page 40). Topping the salad with a high-quality dressing made from cold-pressed oils will add essential fatty acids and antioxidants. You'll find recipes for dressings starting on page 251.

Eat a raw energy bar each day. Raw energy bars are an easy way to pack nutrition in a convenient form. I make a big batch every few weeks and store them either in the refrigerator or freezer. You'll find they are part of the Thrive Diet's daily meal plan.

Eat a substantial, balanced afternoon snack. A properly balanced snack that contains ample protein, high-quality fats, and fiber will provide you with energy and mental clarity. It will supply the nutrition that the body requires and ensure that hunger is not too ferocious at dinnertime. Being too hungry at dinner is a common reason for extra weight gain: People simply eat too big a meal in the evening. A healthier approach is to space out food intake throughout the day.

At a Glance

- A holistic approach is the key element to long-term health and success.
- High net-gain foods reduce energy expenditure and therefore uncomplementary stress.
- Great gains in both physical and mental health can be made by simply eating natural whole foods.
- Fatigue and biological debt can be eradicated by nourishing the adrenal glands. The 12-Week Meal Plan is designed to lower nutritional stress, and lower stress means healthier adrenal glands.
- Recalibrating will yield everlasting energy.
- For permanent results, allow your body to adapt gradually to a new eating plan.
- The Thrive Diet is not about perfection or idealism, it's about progress.

three

the thrive diet for a healthy environment

the energy requirements of food production

The production, processing, and delivery of food have tremendous impact on our environment—greater than any other industry. The energy used in producing and distributing food accounts for roughly 60 percent of the total energy North Americans produce. Of that 60 percent, more than 85 percent is generated from the burning of fossil fuels—coal, oil, and natural gas. The combustion of fossil fuel to create energy in turn creates greenhouse gases. It is now commonly accepted among climatologists and other experts that greenhouse gases contribute to global warming. With the rising environmental cost of extracting and burning oil, not to mention its cost in dollars, the search for alternative energy sources is on.

Although there are alternatives that may help marginally reduce our dependence on oil over the coming years, no great savior is in sight. Ethanol, derived from corn, is a renewable resource and an oil alternative; however, large tracts of land are needed to grow the corn that would yield only a trivial energy gain in the form of ethanol. Even if all the arable fields in North America were planted with corn to produce ethanol, that ethanol would replace only one-fifth of the oil we currently consume. Of course, if fields are dedicated to ethanol production, they cannot also be used to produce food. Simply put, the energy cycle of ethanol is quite high, only marginally lower than that of oil when it is extracted, processed, and refined.

The term *energy cycle* refers to the amount of total energy used to produce any given object, and it is the prime consideration in our search for alternative fuel sources. The goal is simple: net gain. Just as it is in our best interest to eat foods with a high net gain in order to gain maximum energy, the production of food should adhere to the rules of efficiency—more energy should be drawn from the fuel than was used to produce it. This is logical, yet the processing of fuel sources is a tremendous energy draw, so much so that there is not always net energy gain. Some alternatives that have been experimented with have experienced a net loss, not making them a viable alternative.

Food production, processing, and delivery are the greatest threats to environmental health.

Many experts believe that the production of food uses more energy than it returns. One report suggests that for every 10 calories of fossil fuel energy burned in food production, only 1 calorie of food energy is produced. This has many food producers and environmentalists concerned. If food production uses more energy than it produces, it is only a matter of time before resources, namely fossil fuels, run dry. And aside from the possibility of a shortage of fossil fuel, its conversion to energy creates pollution. This study, however, is based on standard agriculture, which includes the raising of animals for food—making this type of agriculture up to 30 percent less efficient than plant-based crop production. The latter is still a strain on resources, but a considerably smaller one. Each time a plant-based meal is eaten instead of a meat-containing one, fewer resources are being consumed. By following the Thrive Diet, you will be helping reduce oil usage simply by consuming foods that require less energy to produce.

Scientists agree that until a new, clean source of high net-gain energy is found, each of us can make a substantial difference by reducing our dependence on oil. Since food production is the largest energy draw in North America, it's also the best place to start: Less processing is better not just from a health standpoint but from an environmental standpoint. The first and easiest way to do this is to simply reduce the number of steps involved in the production of food—from the time it's planted to the time you take a bite. If more milling, heating, and refining are required before food is consumable, more energy will have gone into its production.

Another major consideration in any such discussion of energy conservation is the shift of energy. Each time energy is transferred from one form to another, there is great loss: Energy transfer is extremely inefficient. Throughout our ecosystem, energy is transferred from plant to herbivore to carnivore. With each transaction, a large amount of that form of energy dissipates. It is estimated that each transfer is only about 5 to 20 percent efficient, meaning that 80 to 95 percent of the energy is lost to the environment, mostly as heat. This means that if a person eats a plant, depending on its digestibility and net gain, up to only about 20 percent of the energy within that plant will be passed on to the person to use as fuel or rebuild body tissue. If an animal were to eat the plant, a similar energy loss would take place. If a human were to then eat that animal, another 80 to 95 percent of the energy will be lost. Therefore, feeding plants to animals, only to then eat the animal, is not energy efficient. The draw on oil to fuel those extra steps is significant. In fact, the amount of oil North

Americans consume could be reduced by up to 30 percent if we were all to eat an energy-efficient diet.

protein production: a significant environmental strain

Traditionally, protein-rich foods have taken the most resources to produce, requiring the most land, the most water, and the most energy. Traditional protein-rich crops consist of animal products: meat and milk. Land must be used to grow the food to feed the animal, and pasture land is needed to raise the animal. From there, the processing and distribution of animal products are labor (therefore energy) intensive.

Most standard crops, such as wheat and corn, produce very little protein. What is needed is a plant with a high protein content, enabling it to be fed directly to humans without having to pass through numerous energy-intensive steps to convert it to a reliable form of protein. Fortunately, that plant does exist: hemp. Hemp is both nutritionally and environmentally superior to most plants. Its seed, of which approximately 35 percent is protein, delivers numerous nutrients. And unlike many crops, hemp can be grown in both hot and cold climates. Because it grows much faster than many traditional crops, the harvesting cycle of hemp is shorter, allowing more to be produced in the same amount of time. Naturally resistant to most pests, hemp crops can be grown efficiently without herbicides and pesticides.

In Canada, Japan, and Europe, hemp crops have been planted in over-farmed fields to rejuvenate the soil. (It is illegal to grow hemp in the United States.) Once the hemp has gone through its growing cycle, usually about three months, it is plowed into the soil and left to decompose. After a few rotations, the soil can be used for growing less productive crops. Hemp can thrive in arid conditions, making irrigation unnecessary and therefore conserving water. Since much of the water used to irrigate crops is far from pure, the risk of health concerns arising from irrigation is lower with hemp crops. And finally, in contrast to the protein sources of the standard North American diet, plant-based sources, and hemp in particular, have low oil requirements for their production.

Other primary-source protein foods include legumes, seeds, and pseudograins. I explain each in detail in Chapter 5.

With the current price of oil, how is it that some foods requiring so much energy to be produced are still inexpensive to buy in the supermarket? Farming subsidies, still in place in many countries, including the United States and Canada, shelter us from the cost of food production. If the price we paid for our food were a true reflection of the resources that went into its production, the cost of inefficiently produced food would be sky-high. With the price of oil being what it is, we *should* pay more for food that requires more oil to produce. And in effect we are—since subsidies are provided by the government, a portion of our tax dollar goes into sustaining inefficient food industries.

A plant-based diet significantly reduces our dependence on oil.

soil quality

The soil in which we grow our food is an important factor in its nutrient value. We get many of the trace minerals our body needs from our food. For several of these nutrients, plants are simply the conduit, pulling minerals from the soil. Whether or not these plants then pass through animals before making their way to our diet, the starting point is always the same—the earth.

Organic farmers have been aware of soil value for centuries, even before they were known as "organic" farmers. Once too great a demand was placed on the soil, by too many crops grown without a field rotation, for example, it started to produce less vibrant plants—smaller, less colorful, and less flavorful crops that lacked the healthful qualities their counterparts grown in rich soil possessed. And so the farmers began to enrich the soil. Using decomposing plant waste in the form of compost was a common way of adding valuable minerals and nutrients back into the soil. Allowing worms to develop colonies within the soil was also a way of improving crop quality. Worms help speed the rate at which organic matter decomposes and enable a new crop to be planted sooner. These methods are still used today by some organic farmers. Most of the large food-producing companies, however, take less care in nourishing the soil. Instead, they focus on the plant, making sure it is not harmed by disease or insects, and so plants are sprayed with herbicides and pesticides, which, ironically, cause their quality to suffer. This manner of farming is perpetuated by the increased demand to produce food regardless of nutrient value. The vast majority of these crops are feed for animals being produced for food themselves. Again, passing food through these extra steps is a large energy draw, as well as inefficient use of land.

why the thrive diet is less demanding on the environment

A diet consisting of food that has been minimally processed and consists of primary-source nutrition is less demanding on the environment. Primary-source nutrition means eating solely plant-based foods. As I noted earlier, without adding the extra step of feeding plants to animals and then eating the animal, as is the basis of the typical North American diet, a considerable amount of energy is conserved, about 30 percent—and 30 percent is huge. When energy gains measured in the 1 and 2 percent range are considered "significant," 30 percent is massive.

Imagine if North America reduced its energy usage by 30 percent? If every North American were to eat a diet based on primary nutrition, that is exactly what would happen.

The Thrive Diet is an environmental friendly diet. It calls for eating many foods in their natural state, with little preparation. These foods consist entirely of primary sources of nutrition—plants.

what can we do?

Money greases the wheels of our cultural machine; therefore, it is the greatest initiator of change. We simply have to use the power of economics to help ourselves. To not support corporations that practice poor environmental policies such as unsustainable and inefficient land use, use of toxic herbicides and pesticides, and destruction of old-growth forests is only half the solution. We as informed consumers hold the power.

Smaller, environmentally conscious companies are beginning to attract more and more informed customers each year. Supporting these companies is twice as effective as simply not buying from those whose practices are destructive. For example, to buy non–genetically modified hemp foods grown without pesticides or herbicides puts money toward promoting a clean, sustainable industry. If these sustainable industries are able to flourish because of our support, others will see the economic carrot of "green" agriculture, and they will follow. This is one problem that we can eat ourselves out of.

At a Glance

- When we bite into food, part of the environment becomes part of us.
- More fossil fuel is burned in the production, processing, and delivery of food than in any other industry.
- The more energy used to produce food, the more greenhouse gases created.
- As individuals, the single greatest thing that we can do to preserve environmental health is to base our diet on primary-source foods.
- Simply by changing our eating habits we can significantly reduce pollution, and in doing so improve our health and the health of generations to come.
- Supporting companies that have environmental consciousness will help make their standards the new benchmark of food production.

four

exercise for lifelong health

It is possible to grow a younger body. A younger body is simply one that has regenerated its cells more recently. The key to developing or maintaining a functional, young body is to encourage it to be in a constant state of regeneration. But the body regenerates only if it is given a reason. The best reason comes in the form of regular exercise. Remember, exercise is really nothing more than breaking down body tissue. Once cells are broken down through exercise, the body must grow new cells to replace them. This is an ongoing process. Activity level is largely responsible for the rate at which regeneration occurs, provided that the body has the dietary resources to support it—that it is supplied with premium fuel.

Poor nutrition can convert the complementary stress that exercise provides into uncomplementary stress by virtue of degeneration. Performing strenuous exercise regularly without eating a nutrient-rich diet will speed degeneration of the cells and the aging process. And if the body is not supplied with the building blocks it needs, a stress response will be triggered, causing cortisol levels to rise and body fat to be stored.

How often have you said to yourself, "I did my exercise today; I'll treat myself to a cheeseburger," or, "I've had a stressful day at work—

I deserve ice cream this evening"? People crave junk food during stressful times. But this is when it should be adamantly avoided. Or at the very least, you need to make sure your body also has the necessary building blocks to regenerate after it experiences stress. Immediately following a hard bout of exercise, the body will try feverishly to rebuild what was broken down. At this time, premium nutrition is of even greater significance than usual. For this reason, I have included exercise-specific recipes later in this chapter that will help provide the best possible fuel and building material for active bodies. Providing your body with the best nutritional building blocks after a workout will ensure it continually regenerates muscle tissue. And if nutritionally empty food is eaten later in the day, after the nutrient-rich food, it will not have such a detrimental effect, since the repair process will already be underway. You'll also find that the desire to eat junk food fades if nutrient-rich foods are consumed immediately after exercise.

Exercise has another anti-aging attribute: sweat production. Sweating helps cleanse the pores, which is necessary for skin health. Healthy skin is elastic and supple, giving it a youthful appearance. As you read in Chapter 2, a small amount of direct sun exposure is healthy. Ultraviolet rays in the sun kill bacteria that can clog pores and restrict proper perspiration. And because toxins in the body get excreted through sweat, clear, unobstructed pores allow the body to detoxify fully.

Another benefit of exercise is its influence on the pituitary gland, an endocrine gland in the brain. Soon after you've begun exercising, the pituitary releases a growth hormone that contributes to the building and maintenance of body tissue throughout the body. It also makes losing body fat easier. It has been shown that people who exercise only one set of muscles experience growth throughout the whole body—in muscles they don't even exercise. For example, a person who does squats but no upper body weight training will develop stronger chest muscles. This can be attributed solely to the release of growth hormone. This effect has been shown to occur even when only one *side* of the body is being used in weight training. If a person were to lift weights only with his right arm, over time his left arm would also grow stronger. Not surprisingly, though, the untrained muscles do not develop as quickly as the trained ones. Nevertheless, the exercise instigates body-wide renewal. This is a powerful feature. (Sleep also releases growth hormone, but only if cortisol levels are kept low—as the Thrive Diet aims to do.)

exercise: getting started

We know moderate exercise holds an important position in the creation and maintenance of optimal health. For me, however, it is more than that. Training for competitive endurance sports has been an integral part of my life and a daily routine since I was 15. Because I love it, exercise is relatively easy for me; I never have to force myself. This means the exercise produces less stress, resulting in a quicker recovery than those who have to force themselves to exercise would experience. However, I got to the point where I *needed* to exercise for several hours each day to feel good, both mentally and physically. Luckily, I recognized that this was not mentally healthy—a feeling of dependence never is. I did not want to feel as though I *had* to exercise to feel productive. I began to view it as any other chemical dependency, since that is literally what it was: My endorphins were to blame. Chemicals are released during exercise that improve mood; this can become an addiction of sorts. You may have heard of the runner's high. This is nothing more than a rush of endorphins. One of the biggest challenges for competitive athletes is to not over exercise. In part driven by competitiveness but more because of endorphins, many high-level athletes are in danger of overtraining, and in turn, an overuse injury. Adrenal burnout (discussed in Chapter 1), for example, is a hormonal injury caused by too much stress. One way to exhaust adrenals is to simply train more than the body can recover from.

That said, endorphins can be an excellent motivator. I know most people are not as eager to exercise as I am. I also appreciate that many people downright dislike working out. But keep in mind that not much exercise is necessary to achieve a high level of health. Small amounts of exercise are good for health; larger amounts are good for fitness. The Thrive Diet is about building optimal nutritional health. From there, other facets of health, such as peak fitness, can be achieved if desired.

As little as 20 minutes a day can be enough exercise when just starting an exercise program. A good way to structure a program is to alternate between cardiovascular exercise and resistance training. Cardiovascular exercises such as walking, running, cycling, swimming, and rowing might be done on the first day. Day two might then consist of weight training and calisthenics (using body weight as resistance). Simply alternate days like this, with one day off each week for rest.

Cardiovascular exercise helps develop a strong heart and therefore a more efficient one. The more efficient the heart, the more blood will be circulated with each pump it performs. An efficient heart will be able to pump at a slower rate, which will conserve body energy. The same goes for resistance training: It improves muscular efficacy, making day-to-day activities less physically straining. It also has been shown to improve bone density and strength.

When selecting an exercise, consider your likes and dislikes, and aim to find one that suits your personality. This sounds like basic advice, and it is. Yet, many people participate in exercise programs they don't find enjoyable, slogging their way through their workouts. And as you read in Chapter 1, will power is finite. If you force yourself to do daily exercise that you don't like, it will deplete your will power, making various challenges that crop up in life harder to deal with.

If you want to use exercise to clear your head after a challenging day at work, a run or walk by yourself might be a good choice—if you want exercise to be *your* time of the day, away from others, solo activities are the way to go. If, however, you like the camaraderie and social aspect of exercising, choose an activity such as an aerobics class or circuit training. If you need motivation to exercise, arrange to work out with a friend: Like any other meeting, scheduling to meet a friend for a workout will help get you into an exercise routine and encourage you to stick with it.

There are other considerations, too. Ask yourself if you would like a vigorous activity, such as boxing, or are you more suited to introspective movements, such as yoga? Do you prefer competitive activities to keep you motivated or is competition a turn-off for you? If you flourish with head-to-head competition, try tennis or squash. Do you like team sports? Consider joining a local soccer or ultimate league. Or, if you prefer indoor team sports, check out the local volleyball or basketball court. There are as many activity choices as there are personality types. Check with your local recreation center to see what it offers. You will be amazed at the diversity of activities available.

keep a training and nutrition journal

I suggest you keep a training and nutrition journal to help you stay on track. You might find it inspiring to document your exercise routine in particular. Simply write down what exercise you do each day and how you felt doing it. Include the duration of the exercise and perceived intensity (more on intensity levels below). Also note what you eat each day and when you eat it. Even if what you eat remains the same, the timing of each meal and snack can affect the way you feel and perform. After only a month or two, a pattern will likely emerge. The days that you felt best exercising were probably preceded by the best days nutritionally—a clear indication of the bond between nourishment and performance.

I have kept a detailed journal ever since I began training and racing. It started as both a nutrition and training journal, but then I scaled it down to simply a training journal. Since my diet was so clean, it could be taken out of the equation. I knew that if my performance faltered or improved, something other than nutrition was responsible. I could work backwards from the date of a race and see what I had done correctly to yield a good performance, or what I had done to result in a less than satisfying outcome. It has been by far the best tool that I have had. When I compare a few months leading up to a good performance to a few months leading up to a poor one, what differs immediately stands out. From that information, I know the good points to incorporate and the bad ones to eliminate, and so can design an optimal, tailored training program.

Everyone is an individual when it comes to exercise programs. There certainly is no one-size-fits-all program; if there were, everyone would excel with the same regimen, which we know is not the case. I believe a training journal is of great value, whether you have a coach or not, and even if you are not a high-level athlete. Simply by helping you track your progress and, more importantly, spot those areas where you could improve, a training journal is the best tool for helping you achieve your goals.

proper nutrition boosts exercise's positive effects

The guiding principles of the Thrive Diet are ideal for active people. Efficiency of nutrition—and therefore energy—transfer from food to the body is a key element. As you know, the Thrive Diet began as an athletic performance diet and evolved into an everyday, health-optimizing one. Its fueling and recovery strategies can be applied to any level of activity. Its eating principles will help raise the value of even small amounts of physical activity by quickly aiding cellular tissue repair, thereby reducing biological age and body fat. Properly fueled modest amounts of exercise followed by high-quality nutrition will dramatically increase the effectiveness of the exercise itself, without the need to increase its duration or intensity.

All the recipes in this book are excellent for active people; however, the ones in this chapter in particular are designed specifically for those of you who want to fuel your body to get the most out of your training program. Formulated to be consumed immediately before, during, or after exercise, these recipes have helped me get significantly more out of my training program and have improved my fitness level.

The value of natural, high-quality nourishment is appreciated by the nutritionally savvy athlete: Once the base of general health is obtained, gains in performance can be achieved by tailoring nutritional needs to the specific activity. The timing of nutrition, combined with specifically formulated recipes for athletic performance, is crucial.

speeding recovery

The most important factor for building athletic performance once general health is achieved is recovery. Recovering quickly from exercise is the number one goal of many top-level athletes, for good reason: The closer the workouts to each other, the quicker the athlete will improve. Over the course of a month or so, the effects of quick recovery will be unmistakable in terms of performance gains. Elite athletes aren't the only ones to benefit from quick cellular repair. Speedy muscle recovery is also of great importance for recreational exercisers and even for people who are generally sedentary. If you are able to recover quickly after even light exercising, your body will not have to dedicate as much energy to recovery as it might otherwise need to. This allows other systems, such as the immune and hormonal systems, to remain in better health. Simply put, quick recovery helps conserve the body's resources and therefore energy. As well, the quicker recovery takes place, the less stress is loaded onto the body. It is clear, then, that recovery food, the food eaten immediately after exercise, is key.

Over the years, I have experimented with post-workout homemade concoctions, a whole-food blender drink being my favorite. These smoothies, when next-level ingredients are added (I discuss next-level ingredients on page 217), combine protein, essential fatty acids, enzymes, probiotics, antioxidants, and an array of vitamins and minerals, and contain all the nutrients you'll need for a quick recovery.

Commercial sport nutrition products are not always a healthy option: They are often packed with artificial flavors, refined carbohydrates, denatured proteins, and sometimes even harmful fats. I certainly did not want to consume anything that did not put overall health first. True, some commercial options are not bad; but since I like to know exactly what I'm putting into my body, and keep it completely natural, I opted to make my own. Whole-food energy bars, sport drinks, energy gels, energy pudding, post-workout recovery drinks, whole-food nutrient-dense smoothies, and even performance pancakes are all part of my sport nutrition program.

nutrition before exercise

I'm often asked what the best foods to eat before exercise are. While the pre-exercise snack is not unimportant, its value should be minimal. What I mean by that is, try to ensure that the previous workout was properly recovered from and that the body is so well fueled on an ongoing basis that what is consumed immediately before the workout is not a major factor, fuel-wise.

If you have food cravings—the *need* to eat something—within a couple of hours before the start of exercise, it's a sign that the body is fatigued because its requirements have not been met in the days prior, and it's now asking for nourishment. That being said, it is useful to consume a small pre-exercise snack and to top up energy levels, especially before longer bouts of exercise, such as a long bike ride or a hike.

Being adequately hydrated and fueled before and during exercise will decrease the amount of stress placed on the body, allowing the body to work harder and perform better, and require less recovery time. The body's first choice for fuel during intense exercise is simple carbohydrate. Once the body has burned all the simple carbohydrate available to it, it will opt for complex carbohydrates. It's best to ensure the body is provided with enough simple carbohydrate to fuel activity so that complex carbohydrate is not relied upon. If the body has to resort to burning complex carbohydrate while exercising at a high intensity, it will have to use extra energy to convert the complex carbohydrate into simple carbohydrate.

Eating too much protein before intense exercise will likely result in muscle cramping, since protein requires more fluid to be metabolized than carbohydrate or fat, and cramping occurs when the body is not properly hydrated. Also, protein is not what you want to have your body burning as fuel. Protein is for building muscle, not fueling it. When protein is consumed in place of carbohydrate immediately before exercise, and therefore burned as fuel, it burns "dirty," meaning that toxins are created from its combustion. The production and elimination of toxins are a stress on the body and cause a stress response, ultimately leading to a decline in endurance.

the pre-exercise snack

The most important factor in a pre-exercise snack is digestibility. If the food eaten shortly before a training session, race, or even a routine workout requires a large amount of energy to digest, it will leave the body with less energy—the last thing you want before exercise. Food that is difficult to break down requires more blood to come to the stomach to aid in the digestion process. When blood is in the stomach, it can't be elsewhere delivering oxygen and removing waste products, tasks that must be carried out in order for you to achieve optimal physical performance. And if food has not been digested completely before you begin exercising, you may get a stitch—a cramp in the diaphragm. The more intense the exercise, the more important the digestibility of the pre-exercise snack is.

The ratio of carbohydrate, fat, and protein in the pre-exercise snack is determined by the intensity and duration of the activity. There are three basic levels:

Level One: High intensity, shorter time; activity lasting one hour or less.

Examples: A three- to six-mile run; intense gym workout; game of basketball, tennis, hockey, soccer, or other quick-moving sport that involves lots of intense movement and then rest.

Level Two: Moderate intensity, moderate time; activity lasting between one and three hours.

Examples: Half marathon, marathon, Olympic distance triathlon, intense cycling, power hiking; activities involving more sustained output but less intensity than level-one activity.

Level Three: Lower intensity, longer time; activity lasting more than three hours.

Examples: Half Ironman, Ironman, bike ride, hike, long walk, adventure racing, days spent on your feet in everyday activity.

The intensity of the activity will determine the fuel mixture burned by the body, as illustrated below:

Sources of Fuel During Exercise

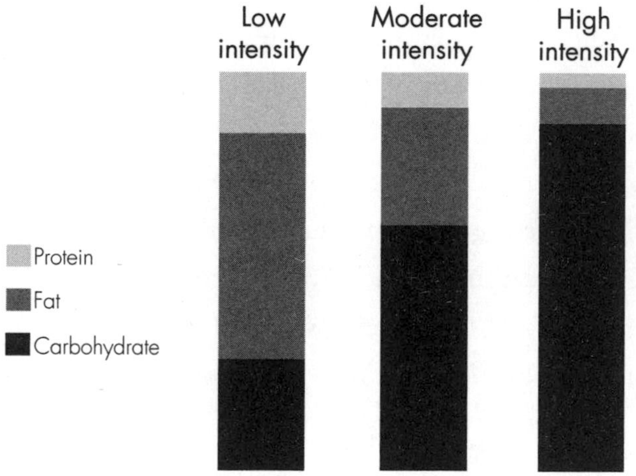

	low intensity	moderate intensity	high intensity
protein	10%	5%	3%
fat	70%	35%	7%
carbohydrate	20%	60%	90%

Source: L. Bravo. Polyphenols: Chemistry, dietary sources, metabolism, and nutritional significance. *Nutr Rev* 1998, 56(2):317–33; M. Colgan. *Optimum Sports Nutrition*. New York: Advanced Research Press, 1993.

The graph on page 110 shows what source of fuel the body is using when performing various intensities of exercise. Of course, everyone's fuel requirements are slightly different, depending on fitness level, diet quality, and, to a lesser degree, genetic makeup. For longer exercise sessions and races, the fitter and better trained the body, the greater percentage of fat is utilized as fuel—preserving carbohydrate stores and in turn increasing endurance.

Level-One Activity. For short bouts of high-intensity exercise, fuel up on simple carbohydrate. The healthiest source is fruit. Dates are a good choice since they are rich in glucose, a simple carbohydrate. Glucose, once consumed, goes straight to the liver for immediate energy; the body does not have to convert it to a different form in order to utilize it. This makes glucose-rich foods the best primary fuel before or during a high-intensity workout. However, it burns quickly, which means that if glucose is the only carbohydrate source, it will need to be replenished about every 20 minutes after one hour of intense activity to keep the body adequately fueled.

Fructose, also a fruit sugar, has a lower glycemic index than glucose, meaning it kicks in at slower rate once consumed, and it burns more slowly, which prolongs its effectiveness. Agave nectar, from the blue agave cactus, is an especially good source of easy digestible fructose. I explain this food in detail in Chapter 5, page 158. Bananas, mangos, and papayas are also fructose-rich (and alkaline-forming). The combination of glucose- and fructose-rich fruit is a very good energy snack, providing both quick and prolonged energy.

One excellent fuel source for high-performance training, racing, or intense exercise that is often overlooked is coconut oil. Coconut oil is a rich source of medium-chain triglycerides, or MCTs. This form of fatty acid is excellent for, among other things, quick energy. As with glucose, MCTs go directly to the liver to be burned as fuel. I explain coconut oil and MCTs in detail on page 144.

I've developed a simple recipe for a snack before a short intense workout or race. Direct Fuel Bites (recipe, page 125), as I call them, combine dates and coconut oil for the ultimate source of quick, natural energy. They provide a direct source of simple carbohydrate. The body gets the fuel from the glucose and MCTs even before the dates and coconut butter are digested.

Level-Two Activity. If I will be performing a mid-range to long workout that lasts up to three hours but is still quite intense, or compete in a race such as a marathon, I slightly shift the ratio of nutrients in my pre-exercise snack. I include a small amount of alkaline protein, usually raw hemp, and a source of essential fatty acids, such as ground flaxseeds or soaked almonds, for prolonged, high net-gain energy. This nutritional premise can be easily applied to any exercise routine, whether as vigorous or not. My raw energy bars (recipes, pages 226–232) and energy puddings (recipes, pages 125–126) supply this ratio. They are digested quickly and supply the nutrients required to sustain high-level performance for an extended period. Simple-carbohydrate based, the energy bars and puddings also provide a small amount of fat and protein to help extend the time between refueling. Including small amounts of fat and protein in an easily digestible form will improve endurance in moderate to long events.

For less strenuous activity, such as long hikes and low-intensity bike rides, a more balanced approach is called for. A good pre-exercise snack in this case consists of about three times more carbohydrate than both protein and fat: a 3:1:1 ratio. Up to one part each of protein and fat for every three parts of carbohydrate can be beneficial before and during longer exercise bouts because, during lower intensity exercise, the body burns primarily fat. This is a critical training zone for endurance athletes, as it teaches their body to become efficient at using fat as fuel, therefore sparing glycogen (carbohydrate stored in the muscle) and resulting in better endurance. However, even a fraction of time spent in the fat-burning zone will burn muscle if not enough amino acids are present, hence the need to consume a small amount of protein before a longer exercise period. Its consumption will slow the release of the carbohydrate, stretching it out for a longer time, thereby improving endurance, preventing muscle loss, and keeping body fat to a minimum.

Level-Three Activity. For those of you who are preparing for events such as Ironman or who participate in adventure racing and other endurance activities lasing longer than three hours, it's important to train your body to become efficient at burning fat as fuel, and in doing so, preserve glycogen stores. Glycogen is carbohydrate stored in the muscles. Within only a few hours of activity, muscle glycogen will be burned up and the body will require more fuel to keep performing at a high level. You will need to eat food high in simple carbohydrate to avoid a decline in performance. However, to reduce the body's dependence on glycogen and the need to consume more food, it is important to teach the body to use glycogen sparingly by shifting its fuel source to fat. Unlike glycogen, fat is plentiful and is near impossible to run out of. Even the leanest of people have enough fat stores to fuel them for several back-to-back Ironman races. The trick is accessing the fat, and this requires the right kind of training. Exercising at a relatively low intensity will tap the fat stores and burn it for energy. A large part of endurance training is spent at a low intensity for that reason, to access fat stores and in doing so improve the body's ability to use fat as fuel. For example, while training for Ironman, it is important to include bike rides that last six hours and longer, to become better at using fat as fuel and depending less on glycogen. The fitter the athlete becomes, the more efficient the body will be at burning fat, allowing the athlete to increase the intensity of the workout while still using fat as fuel. The ultimate goal is to race at a high intensity while burning fat, thereby eliminating the possibility of running out of energy and "hitting the wall."

Before longer endurance workouts, it is important to take a balanced approach to nutrition. Consuming food that provides a combination of complex carbohydrate, fat, and protein will prolong endurance. Before a workout that lasts four hours or longer, I'll eat Performance Banana Pancakes (recipe, page 128). I also eat them before a long hike, walk, or even just a day that involves prolonged ordinary activity.

nutrition during exercise

One objective I set for myself during exercise is to never become thirsty or hungry. Knowing that I'll feel the onset of thirst at about the 20-minute mark, I'll be sure to drink 15 minutes into exercising. During workouts projected to last longer than 90 minutes but under two hours, I'll have a sip of water every 15 minutes. I apply the same method to eating while training. In exercise sessions exceeding two hours, I'll be sure to consume easily digestible nutrients as well, about every 25 minutes. For this, I have developed a number of sport drinks (recipes begin on page 122) and energy bars (recipes begin on page 226).

sport drinks

Sport drinks are one of the sport-nutrition industry's biggest commercial successes. Now as mainstream as many colas, sport drinks are one of the most popular beverages in North America. Making electrolytes and simple carbohydrate readily available in a palatable, easily consumable form, sport drinks serve their purpose. Designed to provide electrolytes to athletes losing them through sweating, sport drinks significantly reduce muscle cramping and spasms, and in doing so improve performance.

Sweat consists of water and electrolytes (electrolytes themselves consisting of several minerals; see Glossary). Simply replenishing water without also replenishing electrolytes can create an imbalance and even lead to a condition known as hyponatremia. Also known as water intoxication, hyponatremia can develop when a person drinks too much water. It is most common among athletes who try to properly hydrate in the days prior to a race yet overdo it and flush electrolytes from the body. Milder symptoms include muscle twitches and cramping; more serious ones include heart palpitations and blacking out.

Because they supply the athlete with simple carbohydrate to fuel working muscles, sport drinks have become a fixture on the athletic scene. Unfortunately, many contain artificial color and flavor and are loaded with refined sugar in an attempt to make them more palatable during intense physical exertion. This, of course, means that drinking them during exercise is actually undesirable. Interestingly, many "sport drinks" on the market are not intended to be consumed during intense exercise: They are simply flavored sugar water, marketed with a sporty image to nonathletic people. The manufacturer's chief concern is making the drink taste good, and the tastes of a person sipping a beverage while inactive are often quite different from those of a person undergoing physical exertion. A light, slightly sour, even bitter taste is often more palatable during exercise, since flavor receptors alter when the body is exerted, and slight tartness is frequently perceived as refreshing. As well, drinks that taste good cold will often taste too sweet when at room temperature or warmer, making many commercial so-called sport drinks impractical.

The concept of the sport drink is an excellent one. The low-grade ingredients in most commercial versions, however, do not equate to excellent functionality—again prompting me to make my own.

Even before sport drinks became popular in North America, a more basic yet much healthier version existed in Brazil. Coconut water, which I discuss in more detail in Chapter 5, page 152, has been used by Brazilian soccer teams for several decades. It has been drunk in many tropical and subtropical parts of the world for centuries. Rich in electrolytes and therefore valuable for the replenishment of those lost in sweat, coconut water can help maintain smooth muscle contractions and energy levels, particularly in hot climates. I base a few of my sport drink recipes on coconut water for this reason.

Another high-quality natural source of electrolytes is found in certain seaweeds. Dulse in particular (see Chapter 5, page 132) has a nicely balanced electrolyte profile. I use dulse in several of my exercise-specific recipes, including the energy bars, sport drinks, and gels.

sport gels

Sport gels are designed to get a high concentration of carbohydrate into the athlete as quickly as possible during competition and training. Their consistency is, as you might expect, gel-like. As is common with commercial products, most gels on the market contain artificial flavors and colors, and their base often does not consist of prime ingredients. Therefore, once again, I opt to make my own. For the gel base I combine glucose-rich dates, blended into a paste, with fructose-rich agave nectar. As I mentioned earlier, the combination of glucose- and fructose-rich foods makes for an excellent quick-energy, endurance-boosting fuel. Designed to be used during moderately intense exercise, these gels digest remarkably easily and get carbohydrate to the working muscles quickly without robbing digestive energy.

athlete-specific recalibration

Another key factor in optimized athletic performance is recalibration. I explain this aspect of the Thrive Diet in Chapter 2. One of the major advantages of the Thrive Diet is an altered "perception" that develops as the body becomes recalibrated. Once recalibrated, the body no longer "sees" food the same way. Recalibration removes stimulating foods such as refined sugars and caffeine from the diet. In doing so, the body adapts to functioning at a higher energy level without depending on foods that stimulate. As an inevitable result, the recalibrated body becomes highly sensitive to any form of stimulation. This means that when you are striving for a greater level of fitness by pushing the body to new heights, consuming a controlled amount of stimulating food can have a useful effect. When the body is spurred on in preparation for a workout with a specific goal—to achieve a yet-to-be-realized level of performance, for example—the stress it undergoes can be considered production stress. Shifting stimulation from uncomplementary stress to production stress will result in greater achievement in the workout. Recalibration, then stimulation, is a powerful performance-enhancing tool and is an excellent tactic before a race or major event. However, to maintain its effectiveness and minimize the risks of adrenal burnout, this can be done only rarely.

One of the healthiest and most effective stimulants before exercise is the South American herb yerba maté. Packed with several trace minerals, vitamins, amino acids, and antioxidants, yerba maté is a nutritional powerhouse. I explain it in detail in Chapter 5, page 157.

You will notice that some recipes have options for yerba maté. These are to be used only once the body has been recalibrated, and even then only on occasion. If you feel that you *need* yerba maté before every workout, it's time to take a rest.

nutrition immediately after exercise

Breaking down muscle tissue on a regular basis and then consuming, without fail, the right nutritional building blocks after the workout is the basis for a stronger, more vibrant, biologically younger body. What is consumed after the workout is vital for cellular reconstruction.

Immediately following a workout, the best snack to eat is one consisting primarily of simple carbohydrate. (A protein "construction" meal should come later.) As I noted earlier, the 45 minutes immediately following a workout is referred to as the fuel window; this window is the best time for the athlete to consume high-quality food. Fed within that window, the muscles will be better able to absorb the carbohydrate in the food, speeding recovery.

A common weight-loss strategy is to restrict calorie intake immediately after a workout. I know many people who will go for a long run, then not eat for several hours, in an attempt to shed body fat. These are the same people who wonder why they feel lethargic during their next workout, and eventually need to skip workouts to feel rejuvenated. In addition to missed workouts, other signs of stress become evident within a couple of weeks. Cortisol levels rise, causing the body to retain body fat and cannibalize muscle tissue, which is certainly not the desired effect.

To speed recovery, the body needs simple carbohydrate to enter the bloodstream—the quicker the better. This means that the post-exercise snack should contain very little fat (even the good kind) and no fiber, since both slow the rate at which carbohydrate enters the bloodstream. For normal everyday activity, a slower release of simple carbohydrate is desirable, and so a small amount of protein is good: As much as 25 percent of the total snack can consist of an alkaline-source protein. Up to one part of protein for every four parts of carbohydrate can be beneficial. This small amount of protein helps speed glycogen synthesis, the rate at which the muscles absorb the carbohydrate. However, a greater amount of protein, in excess of 4:1 carbohydrate-to-protein ratio, will slow recovery.

Immediately following a workout, either a recovery drink or an easily digestible pudding is the best snack. The body often has trouble digesting when it is fatigued (since digestion requires energy, energy the body may not have much of after a hard workout), so liquid and near-liquid-consistency foods are best. You'll find recipes for my Recovery Pudding on page 126 and for my recovery drinks starting on page 127. These recipes contain the appropriate ratio of nutrients. The Recovery Pudding, for example, contains bananas and blueberries, both of which provide simple and complex carbohydrates, as well as electrolytes to replace those lost in sweat. The ground flaxseed and hemp protein supply a small amount of protein, just enough to assist the carbohydrate in the muscle glycogen-regeneration processes. The small amount of hemp oil (or EFA Oil Blend, recipe on page 210) in the recovery drinks helps in the repair of soft-tissue damage, that inevitable by-product of exercise. These foods, especially once blended, are easy for the fatigued body to digest and utilize.

Once an hour has passed since eating your post-exercise snack, it's time for a complete, nutrient-rich meal. Ideally, this meal will consist of high-quality, easily digestible raw protein such as hemp, omega-3 fatty acids (also from hemp and flaxseed), and vitamins and minerals from natural whole-food sources. If the workout was a particularly hard one and you are feeling drained, a liquid meal is the best option. A whole-food smoothie is easier and quicker to prepare than most other complete meals, in itself desirable after an exhausting workout. But, most important, a liquid meal shortly after exercise is of value because the majority of the body's blood will be busy rapidly circulating throughout the body, clearing lactic acid and other metabolic waste from the extremities and delivering nutrients. Remember, the consumption of a conventional meal at this time will require a large amount of blood to travel to the stomach to aid in digestion. Since the blood is needed in the stomach, it cannot remain in the extremities going about its "clean up and delivery" job. With the extra strain of digestion removed by consuming complete liquid nutrition, recovery will dramatically improve.

You'll find recipes in the smoothie section, pages 222 to 226. I also outline there next-level ingredients that are beneficial. Of even greater value after intense exercise and other types of augmented stress, these ingredients will help rebuild adrenal glands, keeping them functioning properly, and speed recovery in general. Or you may choose to use the powder formula I have developed, called the Vega Whole Food Health Optimizer. In addition to the basics, this ready-made smoothie mix contains all the next-level ingredients you'll need. It's available in most health food stores.

I don't classify raw energy bars as exercise specific because they are useful for many types of activity levels. Recipes for these can be found starting on page 226.

The table on page 121 shows the best time to consume selected sports-specific snacks (recipes follow) for maximum effectiveness.

	before	during	after
level one *high intensity activity lasting one hour or less*	Direct Fuel Bites with yerba maté	sport drink	
level two *moderate intensity activity lasting up to three hours*	Energy Pudding with yerba maté raw energy bars	sport drink energy gel Direct Fuel Bites	
level three *lower intensity activity lasting over three hours*	Performance Banana Pancakes	sport drink energy gel with protein energy bars	
any level *to fuel, nourish, and repair*			Recovery Pudding recovery drink

alkalizing foods and exercise

Alkalizing foods are an integral part of the body's post-exercise repair process. If not dealt with, lactic acid build-up from physical exertion, general stress, and acid-forming foods will lead to muscular stiffness, fatigue, and joint pain. If an acidic system becomes chronic, it will show signs of aging and will eventually cause the blood and cellular tissue to degenerate more rapidly than if the system were not acidic.

Athletes in peak training are the most affected by excessively high acid levels (acidosis): Vigorous exercise causes lactic acid build-up, and stress of any kind causes even further build-up. Already physically stressed, many athletes must also deal with various forms of performance anxiety. An increased metabolism, which further lowers the body's pH, is yet another concern athletes face. Combine this with the heftier food requirements of most athletes and the emphasis on protein to aid muscle recovery and you have all the elements of an acid-ravaged body. Following the Thrive Diet will help combat this.

exercise-specific recipes

sport drinks

These homemade concoctions are easy to make and much healthier than commercial versions.

Electrolyte Sport Drink with Ginger

raw option

Especially when served cold, this drink goes down smoothly—a prerequisite of any serious sport drink. The citrus combined with the coconut water and ginger gives this drink a refreshing crispness.

The young coconut water provides the electrolytes, while the agave nectar delivers an easily digestible form of slow-release carbohydrate. The ginger helps minimize inflammation.

Make Ginger Ale (recipe, page 269), but substitute young coconut water for the plain water.

Variation: Substitute lime for the lemon or use a combination of both. Use fresh coconut water, rather than pasteurized, to make drink 100% raw.

Basic Electrolyte Sport Drink

raw option

This recipe is useful if you need a sport drink but are unprepared. It's not as good as the others, but it will do in a bind. Most convenience stores and even gas stations will carry these ingredients.

3 parts of your favorite unsweetened fruit juice (use fresh, not pasteurized, juice to make drink 100% raw)
1 part water
Sea salt to taste

Combine all ingredients in a water bottle or cup.

Mint Carob Sport Drink

raw option

3 dates
2 strips dulse (about 1 tbsp)
2 cups water
1 tbsp agave nectar

cont.

2 tsp roasted carob powder (or cacao nibs to make drink 100% raw)
1 tsp dried mint (or 1 tbsp fresh)
1 tsp coconut oil
Sea salt to taste

In a blender, combine all ingredients; process until smooth.

Variation: Substitute 1 cup young coconut water for 1 cup water to increase electrolyte and simple carbohydrate content.

Makes about 3 cups.

Lemon-Lime Sport Drink

raw

Juice of 1/2 lemon
Juice of 1/4 lime
3 dates
2 cups water
1 tbsp agave nectar
1 tsp coconut oil
Sea salt to taste

Filter out lemon and lime pulp from the juice if so desired. In a blender, combine all ingredients; process until smooth.

Keep refrigerated for up to 2 weeks. Some settling may occur, so re-blend before drinking.

Makes about 3 cups.

fast fuel

These gels can be stored in small plastic zip-up bags and taken with you for long workouts or a race. However, they are easier to handle and consume when put into a gel flask, which can be bought at most running-supply stores. The Direct Energy Bites are a great high-energy snack before a short intense workout.

Add 1 tsp of ground yerba maté for extra kick.

Lemon-Lime Gel

raw

4 dates
1/2 cup agave nectar
1 tbsp lime zest
2 tsp lemon zest
1/2 tsp dulse
Sea salt to taste

In a blender, combine all ingredients; process until blend reaches a gel-like consistency.

This gel will keep for up to 3 days in the refrigerator, but it's best when consumed fresh.

Makes about 3/4 cup, enough to fill two standard 4-ounce gel flasks.

Carob Gel

raw option

4 dates
1/4 cup agave nectar
2 tbsp lemon juice
2 tsp roasted carob powder (or cacao nibs to make gel 100% raw)
2 tsp lemon zest
Sea salt to taste

In a blender, combine all ingredients; process until blend reaches a gel-like consistency.

This gel will keep for up to 3 days in the refrigerator, but it's best when consumed fresh.

Makes about 3/4 cup, enough to fill two standard 4-ounce gel flasks.

Coconut Carob Gel (with protein)

raw option

2 dates
1/4 cup agave nectar
1 tbsp roasted carob powder (or cacao nibs to make gel 100% raw)
1 tbsp hemp protein

cont.

1 tbsp coconut oil

1 tbsp lemon juice

1 tsp lemon zest

Sea salt to taste

In a blender, combine all ingredients; process until blend reaches a gel-like consistency.

This gel will keep for up to 3 days in the refrigerator, but it's best when consumed fresh.

Makes about 3/4 cup, enough to fill two standard 4-ounce gel flasks.

Direct Fuel Bites

raw

These are the ultimate for quick energy. Add 2 tsp ground yerba maté for an even greater kick.

5 dates

2 tbsp coconut oil

2 tsp lemon zest

1 tsp lemon juice

Sea salt to taste

In a food processor, combine all ingredients; process until smooth. Form mixture into a 1/2-inch-thick rectangle. Cut into bite-size pieces. Individually wrap in Cellophane and store in the refrigerator or freezer.

Will keep well in the freezer for up to 3 months, and for up to 2 weeks in the refrigerator.

Variation: Add 1 tsp roasted carob powder (or cacao nibs to make drink 100% raw).

Makes approximately 8 1/2 ounce bite-size bars.

puddings

Energy Pudding

raw option

A nutritionally balanced blend of easily digestible high-nutrient foods, energy pudding is a great pre-exercise snack.

2 bananas

1/2 cup dates

cont.

1/4 cup ground flaxseed
1/4 cup roasted carob powder (or cacao nibs to make pudding 100% raw)
1 tbsp coconut oil
1 tsp lemon juice
1/4 tsp sea salt

In a food processor, combine all ingredients; process until smooth.

This pudding will keep for up to 3 days in the refrigerator, but it's best when eaten fresh.

Variation: Add 2 tsp ground yerba maté for a high-performance version. (Keep in mind that this will also mean greater fatigue later.)

Makes 2 servings.

Recovery Pudding

This pudding is similar to the recovery drinks, simply offering a different texture for variety. It tastes especially good when cold, just after a hot summer workout.

2 bananas
1 cup blueberries
1/2 cup soaked almonds
1/4 cup ground flaxseed
1/4 cup hemp protein
1/4 cup roasted carob powder
2 tsp ground rooibos (grind to a fine powder in a coffee grinder)
1 tsp lemon juice
1/4 tsp sea salt

In a food processor, combine all ingredients; process until smooth.

This pudding will keep for up to 3 days in the refrigerator, but it's best when eaten fresh.

Variation: To further alkalinize plus fortify, and therefore increase recovery rate, substitute 1/4 cup ground flaxseeds and 1/4 cup hemp protein with 1/2 cup of Vega Whole Food Smoothie Infusion or Vega Whole Food Health Optimizer.

Makes 2 servings.

recovery drinks

With approximately four parts of carbohydrate for every one part of protein, these recovery drinks have more protein than the sport drinks, yet less than a smoothie. This is the ideal ratio to help speed recovery immediately after exercise, before a protein-rich smoothie is consumed.

As a variation of either of the recovery drink recipes below, substitute 1 cup young coconut water for 1 cup water to increase electrolyte and simple carbohydrate content. For extra adrenal nourishment, add 2.5 grams of maca.

Lemon-Lime Recovery Drink

raw

Juice of 1/2 lemon
Juice of 1/4 lime
4 dates
2 cups water
2 tbsp agave nectar
1 tbsp hemp protein
1 tsp ground dulse flakes
1 tsp hemp oil or EFA Oil Blend (p. 210)
1/2 tsp lemon zest

In a blender, combine all ingredients; process until smooth.

Keep refrigerated for up to 3 days. Some settling may occur, so re-blend before drinking.

Makes about 3 cups.

Ginger Papaya Recovery Drink

raw

2 dates
2 cups water
1/2 cup ripe papaya chunks

cont.

2 tbsp agave nectar
1 tbsp hemp protein
1/2 tbsp grated fresh ginger
1 tsp ground dulse flakes
1 tsp hemp oil or EFA Oil Blend (p. 210)
1/2 tsp lemon zest

In a blender, combine all ingredients; process until smooth.

Keep refrigerated for up to 3 days. Some settling may occur, so re-blend before drinking.

Makes about 3 cups.

pancakes

Performance Banana Pancakes

These are the best pancakes to eat before embarking on a long workout. They are light and easily digestible, yet deliver an abundance of nutrients to fuel peak performance. Add yerba maté to enhance the quality of your workout—just be prepared to rest longer afterward.

2 dates
1 banana
1 cup Popped Amaranth (p. 209)
1 cup Hemp Milk (p. 268)
1 cup water
1/2 cup sprouted or cooked buckwheat
1/4 cup ground flaxseed
1/4 cup hemp flour
1 tbsp ground dulse flakes
1/2 tbsp grated fresh ginger

In food processor, combine all ingredients; process until smooth.

Lightly oil a frying pan with coconut oil and heat over medium heat. Pour in pancake batter to desired size pancake. Cook for 5 minutes or until bubbles begin to appear in the batter. Flip and cook for another 5 minutes or so. Following the Thrive Diet principle of cooking only at low heat, and since these pancakes contain essential fatty acids that are destroyed at high heat, they are cooked at a lower temperature than traditional pancakes. They therefore take a bit longer to cook.

Variation: Add 2 tsp ground yerba maté.

Makes 2 large servings.

At a Glance

- Regular exercise combined with proper nutrition continually regenerates the body's cells.
- Only a moderate amount of exercise is necessary to create and maintain peak health.
- For long-term success, choose a form of exercise that complements your lifestyle, one that you enjoy.
- Eating the right balance of carbohydrate, protein, and fat as determined by exercise intensity will dramatically improve performance.
- The sport-specific foods detailed in this chapter will help enhance your workout quality and therefore fitness level; these homemade versions are much healthier than most of their commercial counterparts.

five

staple foods for the thrive diet

The Thrive Diet is composed of a number of staples. These are reflected in the Thrive Diet pyramid, on page 40. Although some of the foods central to the Thrive Diet 12-Week Meal Plan are not common in a typical North American diet, most can be found in grocery stores, with the exception of the next-level foods discussed at the end of the chapter. Bigger, more progressive supermarkets may carry them, and health foods stores will almost certainly stock them.

vegetables

leafy greens

Dark green leafy vegetables are a rich source of chlorophyll, important in offsetting stress by alkalizing the body. Chlorophyll also cleanses and oxygenates the blood, making it an essential "modern world" food and a true performance enhancer. Having more oxygen available in the blood translates to better endurance and an overall reduction in fatigue. In their raw state, chlorophyll-containing plants possess an abundance of live enzymes that promote the quick rejuvenation of our cells. The consumption of chlorophyll-rich, leafy green vegetables combined with moderate exercise is the best way to create a biologically younger body.

All leafy greens are healthy; here are some of the more readily available ones:

Beet greens
Butter lettuce
Collards
Dandelion greens
Dinosaur kale
Mustard greens
Red leaf lettuce
Romaine lettuce
Spinach
Swiss chard

dinosaur kale

A large coarse leaf with a blue-green tint, dinosaur kale is a member of the broccoli family. It is rich in vitamin K, folic acid, iron, and calcium. Packed with chlorophyll, raw dinosaur kale is highly alkaline-forming. Dinosaur kale is less bitter than regular kale, and its bigger leaves can more easily be used for wraps. Rubbing sea salt and lemon juice on the kale will soften it, making it more lettuce-like.

fibrous vegetables

Fibrous vegetables are the base of the Thrive Diet pyramid, and the base of a nutrient-dense diet. They include:

Asparagus
Beets
Bok choy
Carrots
Celery
Cucumbers
Daikon
Green beans
Green peas
Onions
Sugar snap peas
Watercress
Zucchini

starchy vegetables

Starchy vegetables are an important part of the Thrive Diet; however, only small amounts are needed. They are at the top of the Thrive Diet pyramid and include:

New potatoes
Parsnips
Pumpkin
Squash
Sweet potatoes
Turnips
Yams

sea vegetables

Sea vegetables, often referred to as seaweed and less commonly as wild ocean plants, have been a staple of many coastal civilizations for thousands of years. Most notably, Asian cultures have long since embraced sea vegetables as an important part of their diet.

Sea vegetables are among the most nutritionally dense foods in the world. Containing about 10 times the calcium of cow's milk and several times more iron than red meat, sea vegetables are easily digestible, chlorophyll-rich, and alkaline-forming. Packed with minerals, sea vegetables are the richest source of naturally occurring electrolytes known. Electrolytes allow our cells to stay hydrated longer, thereby improving endurance—of particular significance for active people—so it's important that we get an adequate amount from our diet.

Dulse, nori, and kelp are the most popular sea vegetables in North America. Dulse provides the perfect mineral balance in a natural form and so is a superior source of the minerals and trace elements we need daily for optimal health.

Other, less common, sea vegetables are agar, arame, kombu, and wakame.

legumes

Legumes are plants that have pods containing small seeds. Lentils, peas, and beans are all in the legume family. Lentils and split peas are among the most commonly used legumes in Thrive Diet recipes for the simple reason that they don't need to be soaked before cooking.

Legumes in general have an excellent nutritional profile. High in protein, fiber, and many vitamins and minerals, a variety of legumes are part of my regular diet. Peas, and in particular yellow peas, have an exceptional amino acid profile. Also rich in B vitamins (in part responsible for converting food into energy) and potassium (an electrolyte needed for smooth muscle contractions), yellow peas are an excellent addition to an active person's diet. Because of peas' superior amino acid profile, manufacturers are now producing pea protein concentrates and isolates. This high-quality vegetarian protein is a good option for people with soy allergies.

Although some people avoid legumes because of their gas-producing reputation, legumes are no more a culprit than many other foods as long as they are prepared properly. After soaking beans and shelled peas in preparation for cooking, be sure to rinse them in fresh water. Rinse them again in fresh water after cooking. The water they soak and cook in will absorb some of the indigestible sugars that cause gas; rinsing it off will help improve their digestibility and minimize their gas production. Another way to improve the legumes' digestibility is to add seaweed to the pot when cooking them, to release the gas. A short strip of seaweed is enough for a medium-sized pot. As with all fiber-rich foods, legumes should be introduced slowly into the diet to allow time for the digestive system to adapt. Gradually increasing the amount of legumes you eat each day will ensure a smooth transition to a healthier diet.

Raw legumes are ideal for sprouting. Sprouting improves both legumes' nutritional value and digestibility—enough so that they may be eaten raw. As well, sprouting allows the digestive enzymes to remain intact, eliminating gas production altogether.

These are the legumes I recommend for their nutritional value and taste:

Beans	Lentils	Peas
Adzuki	Brown	Black-eyed
Black	Green	Green, split
Chickpeas	Red	Yellow, split
Fava		
Kidney		
Navy		
Pinto		

seeds

flaxseed

Of all the plants in the plant kingdom, flaxseed has the highest level of omega-3, an essential fatty acid. Omega-3 and omega-6 are considered essential because the body cannot produce them. Omega-6 is relatively easy to obtain in a healthy diet; it is prevalent in many nuts, seeds, and vegetable oils. In contrast, omega-3 is relatively rare in the plant kingdom, although hemp and walnuts contain some. Flaxseed, however, is the most abundant source of omega-3 (57 percent of their total fat), making it a vital addition to the vegetarian or vegan diet.

Omega-3 is very important to athletes. Aside from its ability to help reduce inflammation caused by movement, omega-3 plays an integral part in the metabolism of fat. A diet with a daily dose of 10 grams (about 1 tablespoon) of ground whole flaxseeds will allow the body to more efficiently burn body fat as fuel. This is beneficial to anyone wanting to shed body fat, but it is of major importance to athletes who need to spare muscle glycogen. As the body becomes proficient at burning fat as fuel (by training and proper diet), endurance dramatically improves.

To understand the significance of omega-3 to exercise, let's compare two athletes, both at an equal level of fitness. One relies purely on his body's ability to burn carbohydrates, while the other has fueled his body with high-quality fats as well. The athlete who feeds his muscles only carbohydrate can store only enough muscle glycogen for about a 90-minute workout. After that, he needs to ingest more or his performance will decline. On the other hand, the athlete who has incorporated omega-3 and omega-6 into his diet (and trained properly) will be able to draw from fat reserves. This means the athlete has a dual fuel source, lengthening the time it takes for muscle glycogen to be depleted while improving endurance—not to mention creating a leaner body.

Flaxseeds are high in potassium, an integral electrolyte for active people, because it is in part responsible for smooth muscle contractions. The body loses potassium when it sweats, so this mineral must be replaced regularly to keep the body's levels adequately stocked. Potassium also regulates fluid balance, helping the body keep hydrated.

Flaxseed contains both soluble and insoluble fiber. Soluble fiber slows the release of carbohydrates into the bloodstream, helping control insulin levels and prolong energy. Soluble fiber, when consumed, gives the body a sense of fullness, signaling its hunger mechanism to shut off. For this reason, people who are trying to lose weight should increase their consumption of soluble fiber. Insoluble fiber is important in terms of digestive system health. Insoluble fiber plays a cleansing role by insuring toxins don't build up and spread to the bloodstream.

Like hemp, flaxseed has anti-inflammatory properties, welcome in any active person's life. Also a whole food, and a complete protein with all essential amino acids, flaxseed retains its enzymes, allowing the body to absorb it easily and then utilize it to improve immune function.

When buying flaxseed, be sure to choose whole flaxseed rather than flaxseed meal. Whole flaxseeds contain all their health-promoting oils, nutrients, enzymes, vitamins, and minerals. Flaxseed meal is what is left over after the oils have been extracted from the whole flaxseed. Flaxseed meal is mostly fiber and is commonly used as filler in baked goods or low-end meal replacements. I suggest buying whole flaxseeds, grinding them in a coffee grinder, and storing them in an air-tight container in the refrigerator. Ground, they will keep for up to three months.

Because flaxseeds are small with hard shells, they will pass through the system undigested if consumed whole. Grinding them exposes their oils and nutritional value so they can be efficiently utilized by the body.

hemp

Hemp foods have been gaining popularity over the past few years, and for good reason. Hemp has many qualities that set it apart from other foods. It is a nutrient-rich whole food in its natural state: There's no need to create isolates or extracts from it. As you read in Chapter 2, hemp in its whole-food state is more alkaline than most proteins, with a higher pH, which is of the utmost importance in keeping the body in an alkaline state.

Hemp's protein is complete, containing all 10 essential amino acids, making it superior to other sources of protein. Essential amino acids are ones that must be obtained through diet, as the body doesn't produce them. Hemp's full spectrum of essential amino acids offers a clear benefit to any active individual. Its amino acid profile helps boost the body's immune system and hasten recovery. Hemp foods also have anti-inflammatory properties, key for speeding the repair of soft-tissue damage caused by physical activity. Edestin, an amino acid present only in hemp, is considered an integral part of DNA. It makes hemp the plant source closest to our own amino acid profile.

I find the digestibility of hemp protein to be superior to all other proteins I've tried. Since hemp protein is raw, its naturally occurring digestive enzymes remain intact, allowing the body to utilize it with the greatest of ease, reducing digestive strain. Because of its easy digestibility and absorption, hemp protein is a good replacement for other proteins, and, in fact, you will need to consume less protein if you choose a high-quality protein like hemp: Quality, not quantity, is paramount.

A high-quality complete protein such as hemp is instrumental not only in muscle and tissue regeneration but also fat metabolism. Protein, once ingested, instigates the release of a hormone that enables the body to more easily utilize its fat reserves, which in turn will improve endurance and facilitate loss of body fat. Because hemp foods are raw, they maintain their naturally high level of vitamins, minerals, high-quality balanced fats, antioxidants, fiber, and the very alkaline chlorophyll.

Freshness is particularly important when selecting hemp foods, including hemp oil, hemp seed, and hemp protein powder. A deep green color, pleasant smell, and sweet, nutty taste are indications of a recent harvest. As with any crop, be sure to choose hemp that has been grown without the use of herbicides and pesticides.

pumpkin seeds

Pumpkin seeds are rich in iron, a nutrient some people have trouble getting enough of, especially if they don't eat red meat. Anemia, a shortage of red blood cells in the body, is commonly caused by low dietary iron or by strenuous exercise. Iron is lost as a result of compression hemolysis (crushed blood cells due to intense muscle contractions). The more active the person, the more dietary iron she needs. Constant impact activity, such as running, reduces iron levels more dramatically than other types of exercise because of the more strenuous hemolysis. With each foot strike, a small amount of blood is released from the damaged capillaries. In time, this will lead to anemia if the runner doesn't pay close attention to her diet. Iron is also lost through sweat.

I always keep raw pumpkin seeds on hand, sprinkling them on many of my meals.

sesame seeds

Sesame seeds are an excellent, easily absorbable source of calcium. Calcium is in part responsible for muscle contractions—of particular concern to athletes. They will need to ensure that they maintain correct levels of calcium in the body. Calcium plays another important role in the formation and maintenance of bones and teeth. Athletes and people living in a warm climate will need extra amounts of dietary calcium since it is excreted in sweat.

I use a coffee grinder to grind sesame seeds into a flour, then store it in the refrigerator, for up to three months. I sprinkle the flour on salads, cereal, pasta, and soups. Several of the Thrive Diet recipes call for sesame seed flour, to increase calcium content. When baking (whether a Thrive Diet pizza crust, for example, or a non–Thrive Diet recipe), try substituting sesame seed flour for up to one-quarter of the amount of regular, glutinous flour called for in the recipe. If the recipe calls for non-glutinous flour, the whole amount can be replaced with sesame seed flour. Since sesame seed flour is slightly more bitter than most flours, you may want to experiment, gradually increasing the amount each time.

sunflower seeds

Made up of about 22 percent protein, sunflower seeds offer a good amount of dietary substance. Rich in trace minerals and several vitamins important for good health, sunflower seeds are a food worthy of regular consumption. Sunflower seeds are quite high in vitamin E and are antioxidant-rich.

pseudograins

As I noted earlier, pseudograins are actually seeds, though they are commonly referred to as grains. Pseudograins don't contain gluten, which makes them easily digestible, alkaline-forming, and suitable for celiacs, who are gluten-intolerant.

amaranth

With its nutty flavor and packed with nutrition, amaranth is one of my favorites pseudograins. Amaranth is quite high in calcium, iron, potassium, phosphorus, and vitamins A and C. Composed of about 17 percent protein, amaranth is particularly rich in lysine, an elusive essential amino acid. Lysine is important for the absorption of calcium from the digestive tract, but it can be difficult to find in plant-based foods, which qualifies amaranth as a worthy addition to a diet for optimum nutrition. In addition, ounce for ounce, amaranth has twice the calcium of cow's milk.

Amaranth consists of about 8 percent fatty acids, found mostly in its germ. Within those fats is a valuable form of vitamin E known as tocotrienol, a powerful antioxidant. With about a 90 percent digestion rate, amaranth is easy on the digestive system and as such is considered a high net-gain food.

With about three times the fiber of wheat flour and almost five times the iron, amaranth flour is a good addition to recipes for baked foods—its inclusion is an easy way to boost nutritional value. But because of its strong, sweet flavor, it is best used as a secondary flour, combined with a primary flours such as spelt or kamut. Amaranth flour also has a gummy texture. Combining it with fluffier grain or seed flours, such as spelt or buckwheat, is a good way to offset this.

Preparation: Cook like rice, at a 1:3 amaranth-to-water ratio, for about 25 minutes. It can also be sprouted (see page 202) or popped (see page 209).

buckwheat

Despite its name, buckwheat is not wheat, nor is it even in the wheat family. Perhaps somewhat surprisingly, buckwheat is related to rhubarb. Containing eight essential amino acids, including high amounts of the often elusive tryptophan, buckwheat is considered a good-quality source of protein. Since tryptophan is a precursor for serotonin (serotonin is formed from tryptophan), having an adequate amount of tryptophan in your diet is important to help enhance your mood and mental clarity. Buckwheat is very high in manganese and quite high in vitamins B and E; it also provides calcium.

When buying, be sure to select the unroasted form. Roasted buckwheat, also known as kasha, is a traditional East European staple. Roasted buckwheat cannot be sprouted and is less versatile in recipes. Because of its mild flavor, buckwheat is easily overwhelmed by the foods it accompanies. Buckwheat flour nicely complements quinoa flour in particular when the two are combined.

Preparation: Cook like rice, at a 1:3 buckwheat-to-water ratio, for about 20 minutes. It can also be sprouted (see page 202).

quinoa

With a light, fluffy texture and mild earthy taste, quinoa balances the texture of other, heavier grains when combined with them.

Nutritionally similar to amaranth, quinoa consists of about 20 percent protein; it is high in lysine and is a good source of iron and potassium. High levels of B vitamins, in part responsible for the conversion of carbohydrate into energy, are also found in quinoa.

Preparation: The preparation of quinoa is particularly important since it is naturally coated in a bitter resin called saponi. Thought to have evolved naturally to deter birds and insects from eating the seed, saponi must be removed by thorough rinsing to make quinoa palatable. Most of the saponi will have been removed before the quinoa is shipped to the store, but there will likely be a powdery residue.

Cook like rice, at a 1:2 quinoa-to-water ratio, for about 20 minutes. It can also be sprouted (see page 202).

wild rice

Wild rice is an aquatic grass seed, rather than a true rice. High in B vitamins and the amino acid lysine, wild rice is much more nutritious than traditional grains. Native to the northern regions of the Canadian Prairie provinces, wild rice is seldom treated with pesticides since it thrives without. (It is also grown as a domesticated crop in Minnesota and California.) Wild rice has a distinct, full-bodied flavor and slightly chewy texture that complements many meals.

Preparation: Cook like rice, at a 1:2 wild rice–to–water ratio, for about 30 minutes. It can also be sprouted (see page 202) or popped like amaranth (see page 209).

fruit

Fruits that are part of the Thrive Diet include:

- Apples
- Apricots
- Bananas
- Berries (blackberries, blueberries, cranberries, raspberries, strawberries)
- Cherries
- Dates
- Dragon fruit
- Figs
- Grapefruit
- Grapes
- Kiwis
- Mangos
- Melons (cantaloupe, honeydew, watermelon)
- Nectarines
- Oranges
- Papayas
- Peaches
- Pears
- Pineapples
- Plums
- Pomegranates

dates

High in glucose, a carbohydrate, dates are sometimes referred to as "Nature's fuel." Upon consumption, glucose is rapidly converted to glycogen in the liver. Maintaining an adequate glycogen supply in both the muscles and the liver is imperative for sustained energy. For this reason, dates are best consumed shortly before, during, or immediately after exercise. Other foods, including chlorophyll-rich ones, convert to glycogen as well, but not as quickly as glucose. The easily digestible, alkaline-forming date is the ideal snack to fuel activity.

I try to use fresh Medjool dates in my recipes because of their relatively large size and small pit. They are available in most supermarkets. However, any date can be used, and more and more stores are stocking fresh or moist dates in sealed containers. If you are using dried dates, you will need to soak them first for about four hours, to soften them. After soaking, they can be stored in the refrigerator for up to one week.

oils

Oils come in a wide assortment, each with a distinct taste and unique nutritional value. The key to keeping the flavors in your meals ever changing and your diet's nutrient value diverse is using various oils.

In the right amount, high-quality, cold-pressed, unrefined oils are among the healthiest of substances. My favorites are hemp, pumpkin, flaxseed, and, for cooking, coconut. Most oils contain the same nutrients as the plant seed they are from, just highly concentrated.

Not all oils are equal. Low-quality manufactured oil is one of the most damaging foods that can be consumed, eclipsing even refined carbohydrate. Many cheaper store-bought baked or fried products, such as muffins, chips, and cakes, contain trans fat, a near poisonous substance unusable by the body. Trans fat, also known as trans-fatty acid, is added to many mass-produced commercial products to extend their shelf life, improve moisture content, and enhance flavor.

As for the oils used in the Thrive Diet recipes, it's important to know which can be heated safely and which are best consumed raw. I never fry with hemp, flaxseed, or pumpkin seed oil because of their low burning point—the temperature point at which oil becomes molecularly damaged. Exceeding the burning point can convert healthy oils into trans-fatty acids. When baking with ingredients that contain fatty acids, such as flaxseed and other milled seeds, it is important that the temperature not exceed 350°F. I rarely bake anything at temperatures above 300°F, to ensure the fatty acids retain their nutritional value. For stir-frying, when the temperature is likely to exceed 350°F, I use only coconut oil.

coconut oil

Coconut oil is produced by pressing the meat of the coconut to remove the fiber. This is the only fat I use for frying. Sometimes called coconut butter since it's solid at a temperature below about 80°F, coconut oil can be heated to a high temperature without converting to a trans fat. Surprisingly, coconut oil does not have a strong coconut taste, and it has almost no smell. When used in cooking, any remaining hint of the coconut taste leaves, making it a versatile oil.

Coconut oil is rich in medium-chain triglycerides, or MCTs. MCTs are unique in that they are a form of saturated fat, yet have several health benefits. The body utilizes them differently from fat that does not contain MCTs. Their digestion is near effortless and, unlike fat that does not contain MCTs (which gets stored in the cells), MCTs are utilized in the liver. Within moments of MCTs being consumed, they are converted by the liver to energy.

Coconut oil and dates are the base ingredients for my Direct Fuel Bites (see page 125), which I eat during an intense workout or race. Also, because of their "direct burn" properties, MCTs are much easier on the pancreas, liver, and digestive system than are fats that do not contain MCTs. MCT-rich coconut oil is becoming the fat of choice for those intent on achieving or maintaining a lean frame.

extra-virgin olive oil

"Extra-virgin" means that the oil is from the first pressing of the olive. The subsequent pressing is referred to as virgin, the one following that produces regular olive oil. With a light taste and color, extra-virgin olive oil is a healthy addition to sauces, dips, and dressings. Although extra-virgin olive oil is a healthy oil, it delivers only minimal amounts of omega-3.

flaxseed oil

As you would expect, flaxseed oil is obtained by pressing flaxseed. Milder in taste than hemp and pumpkin seed oils, flaxseed oil contains the highest amount of omega-3 in comparison to omega-6, at a 5:1 ratio.

hemp oil

Obtained by pressing hemp seed, hemp oil is one of the healthiest oils available. Dark green with a smooth creamy texture and mild nutty flavor, hemp oil is an excellent base for salad dressings. Hemp oil is unique in that it has the ideal ratio of omega-6 and omega-3 fatty acids.

pumpkin seed oil

Pumpkin seed oil is a deep green color with a hint of dark red. With a distinct, robust flavor, pumpkin seed oil is packed with essential fatty acids and has been linked to improved prostate health.

nuts

almonds

The almond is one of the most popular nuts in North America. Almonds are resistant to mold without being roasted, making them a perfect nut to soak and eat raw. Particularly high in vitamin B2, fiber, and antioxidants, almonds have one of the highest nutrient levels of all nuts. That combined with their high level of digestibility, especially when soaked, makes them a worthy addition to your diet. Although almonds don't *need* to be soaked, soaking makes them more nutritious—in this pre-sprouting state, their vitamin levels increase and the enzyme inhibitors are removed, making them even more efficiently digested. Nuts can be soaked in batches and kept for up to a week in the refrigerator (see page 202).

macadamia nuts

Macadamia nuts contain omega-7 and omega-9 fatty acids. While these are nonessential fatty acids, meaning the body produces them, their inclusion in the diet has been linked to positive health benefits. Blending soaked macadamia nuts results in a creamy spread that makes for a healthy alternative to butter or margarine. Although soaked macadamia nuts are recommended for any of my recipes calling for macadamia nuts, they don't need to be soaked if you're short of time or unprepared.

walnuts

Walnuts are rich in B vitamins and possess a unique amino acid profile. Also rich in potassium and magnesium, walnuts can help maintain adequate electrolyte levels in the body, prolonging hydration. As with almonds and macadamia nuts, soaking improves their nutrition and digestibility. Walnuts complement many meals and snacks.

other thrive diet nuts

The nuts listed below all offer high levels of nutrition in a compact form. These nuts can be substituted in recipes for the more common nuts such as almonds and macadamia. Because of their diversity, incorporating them into your diet will ensure a greater variety of taste and nutrition. However, these nuts may not be readily available in grocery stores.

- Brazil nuts
- Cashews
- Filberts
- Hazelnuts
- Pecans
- Pine nuts
- Pistachios

Hazelnut trees grow wild in Europe and Asia. A staple in early humans' diet, hazelnuts have been eaten for thousands of years. Filberts are a variety of hazelnut that are cultivated, and are often produced larger than wild hazelnuts to increase crop yield. Wild hazelnuts and filberts are nutritionally similar; both are excellent sources of the minerals manganese, selenium, and zinc.

grains

brown rice

A staple of many countries, rice is one of the most consumed foods in the world by volume. Since brown rice has been unaltered over the years, the possibility of it causing an allergic reaction is low. Brown rice has a mild, nutty flavor.

The processing of brown rice is far less extensive than that of white rice, making it nutritionally superior to its white counterpart. Since only its outermost layer, the hull, is removed, brown rice retains its nutritional value. Brown rice is very high in manganese and contains large amounts of selenium and magnesium. It is a good source of B vitamins as well.

Purple sticky rice, or Thai black rice, is a nice alternative to standard brown rice. It can be substituted for brown rice at a 1:1 ratio.

To add extra flavor and nutrition to rice when cooking, add 1 teaspoon of rooibos leaves for each cup of uncooked rice.

Preparation: Cook at a 1:2 rice-to-water ratio. Put rice and water in a pot. Cover and bring to a boil. Once boiling, reduce heat to a simmer; simmer for 45 minutes. Remove from the stove and stir. Let cool.

millet

Millet is one of the most easily digested grains. It is gluten-free and its digestion creates a slight alkalizing effect in the body. Probably also the most versatile grain, millet can be either creamy or fluffy, depending on how long it's cooked.

High in B vitamins, magnesium, and the essential amino acid tryptophan, millet is nutritionally dense and complements many meals. Millet flour, with its mild, easily influenced flavor, adds nutritional variety to recipes.

Preparation: Cook like rice, at a 1:3 millet-to-water ratio, for about 35 minutes. It can also be sprouted.

spelt

Referred to as an ancient grain, meaning that it has not been altered over time by either primitive crossing techniques or modern genetic modification, spelt has a long history. Spelt is rich in energy-producing B vitamins and has 30 percent more protein than standard whole wheat. Spelt does contain gluten but in considerably smaller quantities than whole wheat. Because of its gluten content, spelt flour can be used to bind other grain and seed flours in baking. For this reason, and because spelt takes longer than most grains to prepare, spelt flour is the most useful form of this grain. Spelt has a mild, slightly nutty flavor.

Preparation: Soak spelt overnight, then cook like rice, in a 1:3 spelt-to-water ratio, for about 1 hour. It can also be sprouted.

teff

Teff is a mineral-rich grain. Along with its large amounts of calcium, magnesium, boron, copper, phosphorus, and zinc, teff has about twice as much iron as whole wheat. This tiny grain becomes creamy when cooked; reduce cooking time for a slightly crunchy texture. Teff has a slight molasses taste, adding flavor when combined with other grain and seed flours.

Preparation: Cook like rice, at a 1:4 teff-to-water ratio, for about 15 minutes. It can also be sprouted.

next-level foods

Next-level foods are foods that offer a host of benefits above and beyond those in a standard healthy diet. They provide more nutritionally than simply their food value: Because they are easy to digest and have a neutral or high pH, they can help reduce inflammation, boost the immune system, and speed recovery. They are packed with vitamins, minerals, and other health-promoting properties. However, because they are less common foods, you may have difficulty finding them in all stores; health food stores and larger supermarkets will carry them, and they may be fairly expensive. While next-level foods are not necessary to consume as part of the Thrive Diet, they are a good addition to any eating plan, especially when you are feeling rundown. By following the Thrive Diet 12-Week Meal Plan, you will reap the benefits of healthy eating; these foods simply offer additional support.

açaí

Most noted for their exceptionally high antioxidant level, açaí berries are native to the Amazon. Similar to blueberries in size and texture, açaí berries have a deep purple tint. Also rich in essential fatty acids and fiber, these berries are slightly more protein rich than most. Trace mineral levels are high and phytonutrients are rich. In North America, the most common form of açaí is as powder or in frozen packs. The powder is ideal for adding to pancakes, mixing with juice and nut milks or adding to smoothies. Frozen açaí packs can be eaten as a more nutritious alternative to frozen juice bars or substituted for the fruit component of a smoothie.

chlorella

One of the finest superfoods in nature is chlorella, a single-celled freshwater microscopic green algae. I could write a whole book just on chlorella's amazing attributes and practical applications. Capable of reproducing itself four times every 24 hours, chlorella is the fastest growing plant on earth. It also contains more chlorophyll and nucleic acids (DNA and RNA) than any other known plant. It's no surprise that chlorella is the number one food supplement in land-scarce Japan, where it is used regularly by 10 million people.

Chlorella is being investigated in the West as a "land saver." Its amazing rate of growth has made it a subject of study for scientists who aim to improve yields of food-producing land. Chlorella is 65 percent protein, making it by far the most environmentally efficient method of protein production. Contrast this to whey protein, for which grazing land is needed for the cattle and farm land is needed to grow grain to feed the cows; the cows must then be milked, the whey extracted from the milk, the protein extracted from the whey, and so on—all a draw on resources. Plus, since chlorella has the highest level of chlorophyll of any organism, the protein remains alkaline, thus speeding recovery from daily wear and tear and after exercise.

Chlorella is a complete food; it can also be considered a vitamin and mineral supplement. Nutritionally, chlorella is a true superfood, containing a high amount of protein, essential fatty acids, and a plethora of vitamins, minerals, and enzymes. As well, chlorella contains the elusive (at least, in the plant kingdom) vitamin B12, which is extremely difficult for vegetarians to find in forms other than manufactured tablets. Chlorella provides it, naturally.

Chlorella possesses 19 amino acids. Among them are all 10 of the essential ones (those that must be obtained through diet; the body cannot manufacture them). Therefore, chlorella is a complete protein. These amino acids, in conjunction with naturally occurring enzymes, are the most easily absorbed and utilized form of protein. The ease with which these amino acids can be utilized means this is an easy task for the body. Many other complete proteins are much more energy intensive to digest.

So complete is this wonder-food that, when consuming nothing other than chlorella, human life can be sustained for an extended period. This was discovered by NASA when the space agency was looking at ways to sustain astronauts for space travel.

Chlorella's detoxification properties, another key component of the plant, has recently garnered attention in the West. As we know all too well, our air and water quality is declining, and there really is no practical way to avoid our exposure to it. I choose chlorella as a daily body detoxifier. It helps reduce stress on the system from environmental pollutants. At times, I have no choice but to ride my bike on streets with heavy traffic, en route to more suitable training grounds, meaning I must pass through polluted air. Chlorella helps reduce cellular damage caused by free radicals produced by vehicle emissions.

Daily consumption of chlorella is a perfect example of a preventative measure to build better health via a stronger body. Directly enhancing the immune system at a cellular level, chlorella treats the *cause* of any possible breach—as opposed to fighting the onset of sickness (as is all too often done with pharmaceutical drugs).

Nucleic acids (RNA and DNA) and chlorella growth factor (CGF), a compound exclusively found in chlorella, are further attributes that set chlorella apart. CGF is responsible for chlorella's unprecedented ability to quadruple every day. By consuming chlorella, we can benefit from its growth factor. It speeds cell regeneration, slows signs of aging, enhances healing, and expedites muscle recovery. CGF is even capable of stimulating tissue repair when the body's healing sources are overworked because of incessant stress. CGF is capable of swinging the body's immune function north of the proverbial fine line during times of unrelenting stress, thus helping you avoid getting sick.

A CGF of 3 percent growth is considered high; however, most packaging labels don't state the CGF. When selecting chlorella, look for high levels of protein and chlorophyll; some brands do state this on the label. For protein, 65 to 70 percent is considered high; for chlorophyll, 6 to 7 percent.

Since chlorella is a whole food, I suggest a daily dose of at least 1.5 grams (about 1/2 teaspoon); 2.5 grams (1 teaspoon) daily is significantly better. You can't take too much chlorella: Because it is not stored in the body, toxicity is not a risk. However, its full cleansing effect will likely be felt with 2.5 grams (1 teaspoon) a day. I consume up to 7.5 grams (1 tablespoon) a day during heavy training, with a notable improvement in my performance. Some people take up to 15 grams (2 tablespoons) a day to add more protein to their diet. However, since chlorella contains iron, those on a low-iron diet should not exceed 10 grams (4 teaspoons) a day.

coconut

Coconut water is the cloudy liquid inside a coconut. It has a sweet and distinctly coconut flavor. Packed with electrolytes, coconut water is the original sport drink. It has been used for decades in tropical regions to keep the body properly hydrated. The coconut meat, the white flesh inside the coconut, is a good source of high-quality fat and trace minerals. Coconut milk is coconut meat blended with coconut water. This white fatty liquid (which is considered a good fat) has the consistency of cream and is a common ingredient in Thai cooking.

green tea

Prized in Asia for centuries for both its nutritional and ceremonial value, green tea is available in several varieties. The variety getting the most attention in North America recently is matcha green tea. With a slightly bitter yet fresh taste, matcha is a potent green tea that is higher in nutritional value than other varieties. The leaves are ground into a fine chlorophyll-rich powder that is exceptionally high in antioxidants.

While matcha does contain caffeine, that caffeine differs significantly from the type found in the coffee bean. Matcha's caffeine is a type that slowly and steadily releases energy over the course of several hours, meaning it won't cause caffeine jitters, as coffee will. In addition, theophylline does not place stress on the adrenal glands as typical caffeine-rich beverages do. There is evidence to suggest that matcha can help restore hormonal balance and therefore be beneficial to the adrenal glands.

green tea seed oil

With a viscosity and color similar to extra-virgin olive oil, green tea seed oil is high in antioxidants and trace minerals. As with all oils, it carries many of the beneficial properties of the plant it is extracted from: Just as green tea has many beneficial properties, so too does green tea seed oil.

maca

A root vegetable related to the turnip and grown in the mineral-rich volcanic soil of the Peruvian highlands, maca is yet another superfood. Maca, a staple of native Peruvians for thousands of years, is an adaptogen. When the Spanish conquistadors invaded Peru, they had tremendous trouble adapting to their new environment: Accustomed to land much closer to sea level, the newcomers now had to adapt to a land that was at an elevation of 11,000 to 15,000 feet. At this altitude, oxygen in the air is less than half of what it is at sea level. The newcomers were physically stressed beyond their limits. Their livestock, also new to the region, exhibited signs of stress as well, eventually resulting in a decline in fertility. Once the animals were fed maca, however, they soon adjusted to their harsh environment. Making the connection, the conquistadors began eating maca too, with similar results.

Curtailing the effects of stress by helping the adrenal glands regenerate, maca is an ideal "modern world" food. I know I have been better able to adapt to physical stress when supplementing with maca. Maca also works to restore the negative effect that stress has on hormonal health. Even a modest decline—or increase, for that matter—in certain hormone levels will impair the body's ability to build muscle and recover from stress in general. An out-of-balance hormonal system is a catalyst for numerous ailments. A prolonged hormonal imbalance will also inducc signs of premature aging and cause excess body fat to be stored.

Again, balance is the key to adapting to physical stress and, by doing so, become stronger. With maca, I'm able to continue training at a high level while maintaining my body's hormone balance: It enables me to more easily adapt to increased training times.

Maca possesses the building blocks or precursors for serotonin. As you read in Chapter 1, the body will often try to self-medicate when it's feeling overwhelmed by stress-induced chemical reactions in the brain. It's at this time that sugar cravings are prevalent—they're the brain's attempt to raise serotonin levels. A diet that includes a daily dose of maca will supply the body with what it needs to curtail stress and construct serotonin, thereby reducing or altogether eliminating sugar cravings and the vicious circle they can initiate.

Sterols are steroid-like compounds found in both plants and animals that promote quick regeneration of fatigued muscle tissue. Maca is a rich source of sterols (see Glossary, page 288). During the off-season, I build my strength and muscle mass in the gym. Strength is important for any athlete, even an endurance athlete, as it improves the efficiency of muscle contractions. I like to start the season with a bit more muscle than I need since it will be whittled down as the year progresses. I've recently experienced exceptional strength gains when supplementing with maca. I've been able to lift more weight than in previous years and recovered faster. It has enabled me to perform more high-quality workouts. Maca increases energy by means of nourishment, not stimulation.

As I mentioned earlier, including yerba maté in the exercise-specific recipes as part of a pre-exercise or race snack will help you achieve a greater level of performance. However, it's a strain on the adrenal glands. Adding maca to a smoothie along with other next-level ingredients is an excellent way to nourish the adrenals after consuming yerba maté.

When selecting maca, choose the gelatinized form. The process of gelatinization removes the hard-to-digest starchy component of the maca root. The result is an easily digestible, quickly assimilated, and more concentrated form of maca. Gelatinized maca has a pleasant, slightly butterscotch taste and dissolves more easily than regular maca. The published human clinical studies indicating maca's effectiveness were all performed using the gelatinized form.

As with chlorella, I suggest at least 1.5 grams (about 1/2 teaspoon) of maca daily; 2.5 grams (1 teaspoon) is even better. Again, I consume more during times of heavy training—up to 7.5 grams (1 tablespoon) daily—with excellent results. Although it's not possible to consume too much maca—it won't accumulate to toxic levels in the body—more is not necessarily better. For most people, 2.5 grams is enough. Exceeding 10 grams a day will not provide any additional benefits.

rooibos

Rooibos, sometimes referred to as red tea, is native to South Africa. With a distinct but not overpowering sweet, earthy taste, its mildness is a pleasant flavor addition to many recipes. The leaves of the rooibos plant are commonly used to make a tea-like infusion. Similar to green tea in several nutritional respects, rooibos is most coveted for its high level of antioxidants and alkaline-forming properties. Unlike green tea, rooibos does not contain caffeine. While the leaf is rich in minerals and trace minerals, most of this value does not transfer to the water when the leaves are steeped. For this reason, I use whole ground rooibos leaves in my recipes, to get full nutritional value.

white chia

White chia is an ancient plant belonging to the mint family. Its seeds are small and round, similar to poppy seeds. With their crunchy texture and mild, nutty flavor, white chia seeds are gaining popularity in North America. Native to what is now Mexico, white chia has been valued and cultivated since Aztec times; today, most white chia is grown in the fertile soil of the Amazon basin in Peru. Partly because of the rich soil in which it is grown, white chia is extremely nutrient dense: Packed with trace minerals, vitamins, and essential fats, it is a sound addition to any diet.

Because of its EFA profile, white chia seeds are most often compared with flaxseed. Both are rich in omega-3. Unlike flaxseed, however, white chia doesn't need to be ground in order for the body to access its nutrition. White chia helps speed recovery, as it consists of about 20 percent high-quality protein and is packed with antioxidants. Particularly high in magnesium, potassium, calcium, and iron, white chia can effectively replenish minerals used in muscle contractions and lost in sweat. It is also high in both soluble and insoluble fiber, which helps sustain energy and maintain fullness. White chia can be used to replace up to one-fifth of regular flour in baking, to add nutrition and crunch, or substituted at a 1:1 ratio for ground flaxseed in recipes. I often sprinkle about a tablespoon over my salads.

White chia is not yet commonly available in North America; however, as its benefits become appreciated, more and more health food stores are beginning to stock it.

yerba maté

Yerba maté is a South American plant whose leaf is commonly used to make a tea-like infusion. Yerba maté is similar to green tea in many nutritional respects. It is rich in chlorophyll, antioxidants, and numerous trace minerals and is a good digestive aid. Since yerba maté contains caffeine, once I have recalibrated, I use it sparingly. As I discussed in Chapter 4, yerba maté is one of the healthiest forms of stimulation. Its effect on the recalibrated body in terms of delivering energy is significant. It is the ideal food to help you "rise to the occasion" in terms of improved productivity and increased athletic performance because it brings on short-term production stress. For this reason, several of my sport-specific recipes call for yerba maté, first ground to a fine powder in a coffee grinder.

Yerba maté is grown primarily in Paraguay. When selecting yerba maté, I recommend you choose one that is either "wild harvest" or has been grown "with" the jungle, rather than instead of the jungle. By avoiding yerba maté grown on plantation-style farms that replaced old-growth forest, you are supporting farmers of wild-harvest yerba maté, and helping prevent the clearing of old-growth rain forest—as long as these farmers' product is economically viable to produce, the land will not be cleared for plantations or other purposes.

additives

agave nectar

Agave nectar comes from the blue agave cactus. The agave plant is a source of national pride in Mexico, where it is predominantly grown. Its nectar is fermented to make tequila. Unfermented agave is an excellent source of easily digestible, slow-release carbohydrate and trace minerals. With its honey-like consistency and light, sweet taste, agave nectar is easy to get down while exercising, making it especially useful as fuel for athletic performance.

Because it consists of about 90 percent fructose—the reason for its slow release—agave nectar nicely complements dates, with their high glucose levels. I combine agave nectar with dates in several of my sport-specific recipes for this reason. Agave nectar is a good choice for a healthy sweetener; it can be used in place of honey or sugar in many conventional recipes.

apple cider vinegar

A bit of an anomaly in that it is acidic, yet upon digestion becomes alkaline-forming, apple cider vinegar adds plenty of potassium to sauces and salad dressings. Made from fermented apples, cider vinegar is considered a healthy vinegar, while traditional white vinegar is not. It also contains malic acid, which aids in digestion.

balsamic vinegar

Originally made only in Italy and aged in wooden barrels, most of the balsamic vinegar consumed in North America today comes from California. As with apple cider vinegar, balsamic has an alkalizing effect on the system. Combined with an oil blend, such as my EFA Oil Blend (recipe, page 210), or with just hemp oil on its own, balsamic vinegar makes a good salad dressing base.

ginger

Fresh ginger is a worthy addition to any diet. Ginger can help the digestion process and ease an upset stomach. I use it in many recipes. Ginger has anti-inflammatory properties and so aids in the recovery of soft-tissue injuries and helps promote quicker healing of strains. I load up on ginger as my mileage increases to ensure inflammation is kept under control.

nutritional yeast

Nutritional yeast is a single-cell fungus grown on molasses. A complete protein and a rich source of B vitamins, nutritional yeast is especially prized for its vitamin B12 content. Vitamin B12 is scarce in the plant kingdom; nutritional yeast provides a reliable source for those on a plant-based diet. Unlike baking yeast, nutritional yeast is not active, meaning that it does not feed and grow once inside the body. For this reason, those who are advised to avoid yeast (usually meaning active yeast) can almost always tolerate nutritional yeast. Because it melts and has a mild cheddar cheese flavor, nutritional yeast is a good flavor and nutritional addition to sauces, soups, and salads.

stevia

Stevia is a herb native to Paraguay. The intense sweetness of its leaf is stevia's most celebrated feature. About 30 times sweeter than sugar, dried stevia leaf contains no carbohydrates and so has no effect on the body's insulin levels when ingested. Stevia has been shown to help equalize blood sugar levels raised by other sugars and starch consumed at the same time. Stevia, as you might expect, is quickly gaining popularity as a natural sugar substitute among those in pursuit of a leaner body. Improved digestion is another of stevia's benefits.

An excellent alternative to manufactured artificial sweeteners, stevia leaf is a whole food, just dried and ground into powder. I add it to many of my foods. Its ability to help regulate blood sugar levels is important for sustained energy. I even add stevia to my sport drink to improve its effectiveness.

six

meal plans for the thrive diet

shopping list

The following foods are needed for about three-quarters of the Thrive Diet recipes. Devise your weekly (or daily) shopping list based on this general guide and, of course, on the recipes themselves.

Fibrous Vegetables

Avocado (considered a fat in the Thrive Diet)

Beets

Carrots

Celery

Cucumber

Dinosaur kale

Garlic

Ginger (considered an "additive" in the Thrive Diet)

Jalapeño pepper

Mixed greens

Onion (cooking, Spanish)

Red bell pepper

Scallions

Sun-dried tomatoes

Tomatoes

Zucchini

Starchy Vegetables

Squash

Sweet potatoes

Yams

Sea Vegetables

Arame
Dulse
Kelp
Nori sheets

Legumes (raw and dried, or cooked and canned)

Adzuki beans
Black beans
Black-eyed peas
Chickpeas
Lentils (brown, green, red)
Peas (green, yellow)

Seeds

Seeds will keep for up to six months if stored in the refrigerator, and for up to three months if they have been ground.

Flaxseed
Hemp
Pumpkin
Sesame
Sunflower

Pseudograins

Amaranth
Buckwheat
Quinoa
Wild rice

Fruit

Apples
Bananas
Blueberries
Dates
Grapefruit
Lemons
Limes
Mangos
Oranges
Papaya
Pears
Pineapple
Plantain
Pomegranates

Oils

Coconut
Extra-virgin olive
Flaxseed
Hemp
Pumpkin

Nuts

Nuts will keep for up to six months if stored in the refrigerator, and for up to three months if they have been ground.

Almonds
Macadamia
Walnuts

Grains

Brown rice
Oats

Flour

Chickpea
Hemp
Spelt

Sweeteners

Agave nectar
Blackstrap molasses
Stevia leaf powder

Vinegars

Apple cider
Balsamic

Herbs

Dried, or fresh when available

Basil
Chilies
Cilantro
Dill
Mint
Oregano
Parsley
Thyme

Spices

Black pepper
Cardamom
Cayenne
Cinnamon
Cloves
Coriander
Cumin
Curry powder
Nutmeg
Paprika
Turmeric

Extras

Brown rice miso paste
Green tea leaves
Matcha powder
Nutritional yeast
Roasted carob powder
Rooibos
Sea salt
Shredded coconut
Tahini
Yerba maté
Young coconut (or coconut milk)

appliances needed

The Thrive Diet recipes require only a few appliances:

- *blender* (I use a Vita-Mix), for making smoothies, soups, salad dressings, sport drinks, and energy gels,
- *food processor,* for energy puddings, pizza crusts, raw bars, crackers, spreads, and burgers,
- *coffee grinder,* for grinding seeds into flour, and rooibos, yerba maté, and green tea leaves into powder.

traveling and the thrive diet

Believe it or not, the Thrive Diet is an easy eating plan to stick with while on the road. It's not uncommon for me to be traveling for several months of the year, and my eating plan has to be functional within the limitations of life on the road. Here are a few tips.

plan ahead

Depending on the length of your trip, you might be able to bring food with you. I sometimes prepare a few batches of raw energy bars, individually wrapping them in plastic wrap. These travel well: They are compact, it doesn't matter if they get a bit squished, and no refrigeration is required. Plus, they deliver lots of energy while taking up only a small amount of space. They can be carried easily with you. I now usually pack a stash of Vega Whole Food Energy Bars (see Resources), which are the commercial versions of the Thrive Diet bar recipes beginning on page 226.

grocery shopping

When I arrive at my destination, I'll do a big shop at the local supermarket. Fresh fruit and vegetables form the majority of my purchases. If a farmers' market is nearby, I'll go to that—some of the freshest, tastiest food I've ever eaten has come straight from the person who grew it. The freshness is unparalleled and being local means fewer resources went into getting the food to the consumer, since the food didn't have to travel a great distance. Don't be deterred if local farmers don't have organic certification, as certification is too expensive for many small operations. Despite this, many of these farmers grow their fruit and vegetables without using herbicides or pesticides.

grazing

Since most people are on the go while on the road, grazing has a definite advantage: You may not even need to take a lunch break, and when dinnertime arrives, a big salad and a vegetable serving will likely be enough.

restaurants

Travel and business often involves eating in restaurants—mine certainly does. There is no need to avoid restaurants just because they can't make you a quinoa beet pizza crust topped with sun-dried tomato marinara sauce and vegetables. Almost any restaurant can make you a salad. In fact, some of the best (the biggest, and with the most seeds and avocado) salads that I've eaten have been while on the road, and from unlikely sources. Ironically, many steak-houses make good salads. If your colleagues or companions are going to a restaurant that you don't think will be able to accommodate your eating style, be flexible. Most restaurants will be happy to load up your salad with extra vegetables, or put together a large plate of vegetables, even if it's not on the menu. Brown rice and avocado will be on hand at many restaurants as well. A bowl of rice, sliced avocado, and lemon juice squeezed on top, accompanied by a salad, is a reasonable meal, and made with common ingredients. Mexican restaurants often have fresh, homemade salsa; try it with vegetables.

I know that I won't be able to get a balanced, complete Thrive Diet–approved meal in most North American restaurants, and that's fine. I simply eat lightly and have a nutritionally balanced smoothie when I return to my room. For these times I use an individual-serving-size pouch of Vega Whole Food Health Optimizer powder (see Resources) mixed with water. It covers all my nutritional bases and is easy to travel with; that's one of the reasons I developed it.

the meal plan

The Thrive Diet 12-Week Meal Plan is structured in such a way that it balances nutrient intake throughout the day. Portion size is not an important factor of the Thrive Diet. Since all the food is healthy and non-stimulating, feel free to have whatever serving size you like. However, since there are three meals and three snacks each day, you will likely find that small to moderate portion sizes are all that you want.

Since the meal plan is based on nutrient-dense foods, it is common to fill up easily; yet, eating more is certainly an option. The Thrive Diet is not a diet of deprivation. If you feel as though you need to eat larger portions, do so. Gaining excess body fat is hard to do on the Thrive Diet. If you roughly stick to the meal plan, large portions of the recipes at each meal and snack can be eaten each day without gaining weight, as long as you are eating at the right times.

Timing of nutrition is an often overlooked aspect of overall health. It is possible to eat all the right food but at less than optimal times, therefore inhibiting effectiveness. For example, a snack high in dense carbohydrate will boost muscle glycogen levels and speed recovery after a training session. Yet, it would hinder the release of growth hormone if consumed close to bedtime. A high-protein meal a few hours after exercise will help repair damaged muscle tissue. Conversely, a high-protein meal immediately following exercise can inhibit proper hydration, leading to prolonged recovery. A sugary snack during an intense training session can improve endurance by supplying the muscles with readily available fuel, whereas a sugary snack eaten while sitting in front of a computer will, within an hour or so, make concentration harder and precipitate fatigue.

The meal plan is meant to serve as a guide only. You can follow it closely, or you can simply incorporate elements of it into your existing meal plan. Of course, the closer it's followed, the quicker you will reduce nutritional stress and improve your overall health. However, even one snack or one meal from it each day will be helpful. Start slowly, including a smoothie each day in your diet, progressing to eating a salad a few times a week, and take it from there. Once you've recalibrated your system, the meal plan will be easy to stick with.

the thrive diet 12-week meal plan

Unless specified, smoothie, energy bar, raw vegetable, and fruit selections are of your choice. For added convenience and increased nutritional value, smoothie recipes may be substituted for Vega Whole Food Health Optimizer or can be made with Vega Whole Food Smoothie Infusion. Energy bars may be substituted for Vega Whole Food Energy Bars.

week 1

day 1

Breakfast: Wild Rice Yam Pancakes (p. 212) with agave nectar and fruit

Morning snack: energy bar

Lunch: Cucumber Pesto Salad (p. 250) with Tomato Basil Dressing (p. 256)

Afternoon snack: smoothie

Dinner: Almond Flaxseed Burger (p. 233) with mixed greens and Sweet Pepper Hemp Pesto (p. 267)

After-dinner snack: Zucchini Chips (p. 260)

day 2

Breakfast: Toasted Apple Cinnamon Cereal (p. 216) with Hemp Milk (p. 268)

Morning snack: energy bar

Lunch: Popped Amaranth Hemp Seed Salad (p. 249) with Cayenne Dill Tahini Dressing (p. 253)

Afternoon snack: smoothie

Dinner: Adzuki Bean Quinoa Sesame Pizza (p. 237)

After-dinner snack: Vegetable Crackers (p. 259) with Sunflower Seed Pâté (p. 266)

day 3

Breakfast: Banana Ginger Pear Cereal (p. 215) with Rooibos Almond Milk (p. 268)

Morning snack: energy bar

Lunch: Spicy Black-Eyed Pea Quinoa Pizza (p. 235)

Afternoon snack: smoothie

Dinner: Cucumber Pesto Salad (p. 250) with Tomato Basil Dressing (p. 256)

After-dinner snack: Crunchy Cinnamon Plantain Strips (p. 242)

day 4

Breakfast: Garlic Oregano Yam Oven Fries (p. 244) with Ketchup (p. 261)

Morning snack: green smoothie

Lunch: Sunflower Seed Beet Pizza (p. 237)

Afternoon snack: energy bar

Dinner: Popped Amaranth Hemp Seed Salad (p. 249) with Cayenne Dill Tahini Dressing (p. 253)

After-dinner snack: Vegetable Crackers (p. 259) with Sunflower Seed Pâté (p. 266)

day 5

Breakfast: smoothie

Morning snack: Green Tea Ginger Lime Crackers (p. 258) with Miso Kelp Guacamole (p. 263)

Lunch: Crunchy Cinnamon Plantain and Macadamia Nut Salad (p. 248) with Mango Lime Dressing (p. 254)

Afternoon snack: energy bar

Dinner: Popped Amaranth Rooibos Pizza (p. 239)

After-dinner snack: Zucchini Chips (p. 260) with Sweet Pepper Hemp Pesto (p. 267)

day 6

Breakfast: smoothie

Morning snack: energy bar

Lunch: Creamy Carrot Salad (p. 250) with Cayenne Dill Tahini Dressing (p. 253)

Afternoon snack: Curry Lentil Crackers (p. 259) with Pineapple Salsa (p. 265)

Dinner: Pecan Sunflower Burger (p. 233) with mixed greens and Sweet Pepper Hemp Pesto (p. 267)

After-dinner snack: Zucchini Chips (p. 260) with Macadamia Dill Dressing (p. 255)

day 7

Breakfast: smoothie

Morning snack: energy bar

Lunch: Dinosaur Kale Quinoa Wrap (p. 241) and Creamy Ginger Carrot Soup (p. 245)

Afternoon snack: Vegetable Crackers (p. 259) with Sunflower Seed Pâté (p. 266)

Dinner: Cucumber Pesto Salad (p. 250) with Tomato Basil Dressing (p. 256)

After-dinner snack: walnuts

week 2

day 1

Breakfast: smoothie

Morning snack: energy bar

Lunch: Lemon Crisp Beet Salad (p. 249) with Orange Pumpkin Seed Dressing (p. 255)

Afternoon snack: Crunchy Cinnamon Plantain Strips (p. 242) with Black-Eyed Pea Cayenne Salsa (p. 265)

Dinner: Dinosaur Kale Quinoa Wrap (p. 241) and Sesame Miso Soup (p. 245)

After-dinner snack: Banana Coconut Pie (p. 270)

day 2

Breakfast: green smoothie

Morning snack: fruit and pumpkin seeds

Lunch: Zucchini Chip Almond Salad (p. 250) with Pomegranate Poppy Seed Dressing (p. 257)

Afternoon snack: energy bar

Dinner: Spicy Black-Eyed Pea Quinoa Pizza (p. 235)

After-dinner snack: Green Soup (p. 246)

day 3

Breakfast: Garlic Oregano Yam Oven Fries (p. 244) with Creamy Nutritional Yeast Sauce (p. 262)

Morning snack: green smoothie

Lunch: Curry Lentil Rice Pizza (p. 239)

Afternoon snack: energy bar

Dinner: Cucumber Pesto Salad (p. 250) with Tomato Basil Dressing (p. 256)

After-dinner snack: almonds

day 4

Breakfast: Toasted Apple Cinnamon Cereal (p. 216) with fruit and Hemp Milk (p. 268)

Morning snack: energy bar

Lunch: Sunflower Seed Beet Pizza (p. 237)

Afternoon snack: smoothie

Dinner: Creamy Carrot Salad (p. 250) with Cayenne Dill Tahini Dressing (p. 253)

After-dinner snack: Creamy Pepper Soup (p. 246)

day 5

Breakfast: Banana Ginger Pear Cereal (p. 215) with Rooibos Almond Milk (p. 268)

Morning snack: smoothie

Lunch: Cucumber Pesto Salad (p. 250) with Tomato Basil Dressing (p. 256)

Afternoon snack: energy bar

Dinner: Popped Amaranth Rooibos Pizza (p. 239)

After-dinner snack: Green Tea Ginger Lime Crackers (p. 258) with Black-Eyed Pea Cayenne Salsa (p. 265)

day 6

Breakfast: smoothie

Morning snack: Curry Lentil Crackers (p. 259) with Black Bean Lime Salsa (p. 264)

Lunch: Popped Amaranth Hemp Seed Salad (p. 249) with Cayenne Dill Tahini Dressing (p. 253)

Afternoon snack: energy bar

Dinner: Pecan Sunflower Burger (p. 233) with mixed greens and Mango Chutney (p. 263)

After-dinner snack: Green Soup (p. 246)

day 7

Breakfast: Buckwheat Pancakes (p. 212) with raw almond butter and fruit

Morning snack: energy bar

Lunch: Zucchini Chip Almond Salad (p. 250) with Pomegranate Poppy Seed Dressing (p. 257)

Afternoon snack: smoothie

Dinner: Zucchini Pasta (p. 243) with Spicy Sun-Dried Tomato Marinara Sauce (p. 266) and Creamy Pepper Soup (p. 246)

After-dinner snack: Crunchy Cinnamon Plantain Strips (p. 242)

week 3

day 1

Breakfast: Garlic Oregano Yam Oven Fries (p. 244) with Green Tea Miso Gravy (p. 264)

Morning snack: green smoothie

Lunch: Sunflower Seed Beet Pizza (p. 237)

Afternoon snack: energy bar

Dinner: Crunchy Cinnamon Plantain and Macadamia Nut Salad (p. 248) with Cucumber Dill Dressing (p. 256)

After-dinner snack: Sesame Miso Soup (p. 245)

day 2

Breakfast: Pomegranate Green Tea Pancakes (p. 213) with fruit

Morning snack: energy bar

Lunch: Cucumber Pesto Salad (p. 250) with Tomato Basil Dressing (p. 256)

Afternoon snack: smoothie

Dinner: Walnut Hemp Burger (p. 233) with mixed greens and Black Bean Lime Salsa (p. 264)

After-dinner snack: Arame Seaweed Salad (p. 251)

day 3

Breakfast: Banana Ginger Pear Cereal (p. 215) with Rooibos Almond Milk (p. 268)

Morning snack: energy bar

Lunch: Ginger Lime Squash (p. 241)

Afternoon snack: Zucchini Pasta (p. 243) with Spicy Sun-Dried Tomato Marinara Sauce (p. 266)

Dinner: Creamy Carrot Salad (p. 250) with Cayenne Dill Tahini Dressing (p. 254) and Creamy Pepper Soup (p. 244)

After-dinner snack: Crunchy Cinnamon Plantain Strips (p. 242)

day 4

Breakfast: smoothie

Morning snack: Lemon Sesame Crisps (p. 260)

Lunch: Lemon Crisp Beet Salad (p. 249) with Creamy Ginger Dressing (p. 254)

Afternoon snack: energy bar

Dinner: Creamy Pepper Soup (p. 246) with Curry Lentil Crackers (p. 259) and Sweet Pepper Hemp Pesto (p. 267)

After-dinner snack: almonds

day 5

Breakfast: smoothie

Morning snack: Crunchy Cinnamon Plantain Strips (p. 242) with Black-Eyed Pea Cayenne Salsa (p. 265)

Lunch: Zucchini Chip Almond Salad (p. 250) with Pomegranate Poppy Seed Dressing (p. 257)

Afternoon snack: energy bar

Dinner: Spicy Black-Eyed Pea Quinoa Pizza (p. 235)

After-dinner snack: Arame Seaweed Salad (p. 251)

day 6

Breakfast: Toasted Apple Cinnamon Cereal (p. 216) with fruit and Chocolate Hemp Milk (p. 268)

Morning snack: energy bar

Lunch: Cucumber Dill Salad (p. 249) with Tomato Basil Dressing (p. 256)

Afternoon snack: smoothie

Dinner: Curry Lentil Rice Pizza (p. 239)

After-dinner snack: Sesame Miso Soup (p. 245)

day 7

Breakfast: smoothie

Morning snack: energy bar

Lunch: Cucumber Pesto Salad (p. 250) with Tomato Basil Dressing (p. 256)

Afternoon snack: Curry Lentil Crackers (p. 259) with Black-Eyed Pea Cayenne Salsa (p. 265)

Dinner: Dinosaur Kale Quinoa Wrap (p. 241) and Creamy Ginger Carrot Soup (p. 245)

After-dinner snack: Banana Coconut Pie (p. 270)

week 4

day 1

Breakfast: Garlic Oregano Yam Oven Fries (p. 244) with Ketchup (p. 261)

Morning snack: green smoothie

Lunch: Sunflower Seed Beet Pizza (p. 237)

Afternoon snack: energy bar

Dinner: Creamy Carrot Salad (p. 250) with Cayenne Dill Tahini Dressing (p. 253)

After-dinner snack: almonds

day 2

Breakfast: Banana Ginger Pear Cereal (p. 215) with Rooibos Almond Milk (p. 268)

Morning snack: energy bar

Lunch: Popped Amaranth Hemp Seed Salad (p. 249) with Pomegranate Poppy Seed Dressing (p. 257)

Afternoon snack: smoothie

Dinner: Spicy Black-Eyed Pea Quinoa Pizza (p. 235)

After-dinner snack: raw vegetables with Caesar Dressing (p. 255)

day 3

Breakfast: Toasted Apple Cinnamon Cereal (p. 216) with Hemp Milk (p. 268)

Morning snack: energy bar

Lunch: Chickpea Curry Pizza (p. 236)

Afternoon snack: Creamy Pepper Soup (p. 246) with Vegetable Crackers (p. 259)

Dinner: Cucumber Pesto Salad (p. 250) with Tomato Basil Dressing (p. 256)

After-dinner snack: pumpkin seeds

day 4

Breakfast: Ginger Pear Smoothie (p. 223)

Morning snack: Crunchy Cinnamon Plantain Strips (p. 242) with Black-Eyed Pea Cayenne Salsa (p. 265)

Lunch: Lemon Crisp Beet Salad (p. 249) with Orange Pumpkin Seed Dressing (p. 255)

Afternoon snack: energy bar

Dinner: Pecan Sunflower Burger (p. 233) with mixed greens and Mango Chutney (p. 263)

After-dinner snack: almonds

day 5

Breakfast: Blueberry Pancakes (p. 213) with raw almond butter and fruit

Morning snack: energy bar

Lunch: Popped Amaranth Hemp Seed Salad (p. 249) with Cayenne Dill Tahini Dressing (p. 253)

Afternoon snack: smoothie

Dinner: Lemon Ginger Plantain with Dulse (p. 242) and Sesame Miso Soup (p. 245)

After-dinner snack: Zucchini Chips (p. 260)

day 6

Breakfast: smoothie

Morning snack: energy bar

Lunch: Creamy Carrot Salad (p. 250) with Cayenne Dill Tahini Dressing (p. 253)

Afternoon snack: Curry Lentil Crackers (p. 259) with Black Bean Lime Salsa (p. 264)

Dinner: Dinosaur Kale Quinoa Wrap (p. 241) and Vegetable Crackers (p. 259) and Sunflower Seed Pâté (p. 266)

After-dinner snack: almonds

day 7

Breakfast: smoothie

Morning snack: raw vegetables with Miso Kelp Guacamole (p. 263)

Lunch: Cucumber Pesto Salad (p. 250) with Creamy Ginger Dressing (p. 254)

Afternoon snack: energy bar

Dinner: Wild Rice Split Pea Pizza (p. 240)

After-dinner snack: walnuts

week 5

day 1

Breakfast: smoothie

Morning snack: energy bar

Lunch: Cucumber Pesto Salad (p. 250) with Tomato Basil Dressing (p. 256)

Afternoon snack: fruit

Dinner: Ginger Lime Squash (p. 241) and Creamy Pepper Soup (p. 246)

After-dinner snack: Zucchini Pasta (p. 243) with Spicy Sun-Dried Tomato Marinara Sauce (p. 266)

day 2

Breakfast: Banana Chocolate Pancakes (p. 214) with raw almond butter and fruit

Morning snack: smoothie

Lunch: Zucchini Chip Almond Salad (p. 250) with Cayenne Dill Tahini Dressing (p. 253)

Afternoon snack: energy bar

Dinner: Zucchini Pasta (p. 243) with Spicy Sun-Dried Tomato Marinara Sauce (p. 266) and Creamy Pepper Soup (p. 246)

After-dinner snack: pistachios

day 3

Breakfast: Toasted Apple Cinnamon Cereal (p. 216) with fruit and Hemp Milk (p. 268)

Morning snack: energy bar

Lunch: Sweet Potato Sesame Pizza (p. 238)

Afternoon snack: raw vegetables with Sweet Pepper Hemp Pesto (p. 267)

Dinner: Cucumber Dill Salad (p. 249) with Pomegranate Poppy Seed Dressing (p. 257)

After-dinner snack: Banana Coconut Pie (p. 270)

day 4

Breakfast: smoothie

Morning snack: energy bar

Lunch: Creamy Carrot Salad (p. 250) with Cayenne Dill Tahini Dressing (p. 253)

Afternoon snack: Green Tea Ginger Lime Crackers (p. 258) with Black-Eyed Pea Cayenne Salsa (p. 265)

Dinner: Pecan Sunflower Burger (p. 233) with mixed greens and Green Tea Miso Gravy (p. 264)

After-dinner snack: Arame Seaweed Salad (p. 251)

day 5

Breakfast: Pomegranate Green Tea Pancakes (p. 213) with raw tahini and fruit

Morning snack: energy bar

Lunch: Popped Amaranth Hemp Seed Salad (p. 249) with Cayenne Dill Tahini Dressing (p. 253)

Afternoon snack: smoothie

Dinner: Dinosaur Kale Quinoa Wrap (p. 241) and Crunchy Cinnamon Plantain Strips (p. 242) with Black-Eyed Pea Cayenne Salsa (p. 265)

After-dinner snack: almonds

day 6

Breakfast: Toasted Apple Cinnamon Cereal (p. 216) with Rooibos Almond Milk (p. 268)

Morning snack: energy bar

Lunch: Cucumber Pesto Salad (p. 250) with Tomato Basil Dressing (p. 256)

Afternoon snack: Ginger Pear Smoothie (p. 223)

Dinner: Popped Amaranth Rooibos Pizza (p. 239)

After-dinner snack: Vegetable Crackers (p. 259)

day 7

Breakfast: Garlic Oregano Yam Oven Fries (p. 244) with Sweet Pepper Hemp Pesto (p. 267)

Morning snack: green smoothie

Lunch: Spicy Black-Eyed Pea Quinoa Pizza (p. 235)

Afternoon snack: energy bar

Dinner: Cucumber Dill Salad (p. 249) with Cucumber Dill Dressing (p. 256)

After-dinner snack: Vegetable Crackers (p. 259)

week 6

day 1

Breakfast: smoothie

Morning snack: Lemon Ginger Plantain with Dulse (p. 242)

Lunch: Zucchini Chip Almond Salad (p. 250) with Pomegranate Poppy Seed Dressing (p. 257)

Afternoon snack: energy bar

Dinner: Almond Flaxseed Burger (p. 233) with mixed greens and Black-Eyed Pea Cayenne Salsa (p. 265)

After-dinner snack: Zucchini Chips (p. 260)

day 2

Breakfast: smoothie

Morning snack: energy bar

Lunch: Avocado Cayenne Salad (p. 248) with Balsamic Vinaigrette (p. 256)

Afternoon snack: Zucchini Pasta (p. 243) with Spicy Sun-Dried Tomato Marinara Sauce (p. 266)

Dinner: Dinosaur Kale Quinoa Wrap (p. 241) with Miso Kelp Guacamole (p. 263)

After-dinner snack: Banana Coconut Pie (p. 270)

day 3

Breakfast: Garlic Oregano Yam Oven Fries (p. 244) with Creamy Nutritional Yeast Sauce (p. 262)

Morning snack: raw vegetables with Cayenne Dill Tahini Dressing (p. 253)

Lunch: Zucchini Pasta (p. 243) with Spicy Sun-Dried Tomato Marinara Sauce (p. 266) and Creamy Pepper Soup (p. 246)

Afternoon snack: energy bar

Dinner: Cucumber Pesto Salad (p. 250) with Tomato Basil Dressing (p. 256)

After-dinner snack: Sesame Miso Soup (p. 245)

day 4

Breakfast: Banana Ginger Pear Cereal (p. 215) with Rooibos Almond Milk (p. 268)

Morning snack: energy bar

Lunch: Cucumber Dill Salad (p. 249) with Pomegranate Poppy Seed Dressing (p. 257)

Afternoon snack: smoothie

Dinner: Sweet Potato Sesame Pizza (p. 238)

After-dinner snack: raw vegetables with Sweet Pepper Hemp Pesto (p. 267)

day 5

Breakfast: Toasted Apple Cinnamon Cereal (p. 216) with Hemp Milk (p. 268)

Morning snack: energy bar

Lunch: Chili Kidney Bean Pizza (p. 238)

Afternoon snack: smoothie

Dinner: Popped Amaranth Hemp Seed Salad (p. 249) with Ginger Carrot Dressing (p. 254)

After-dinner snack: Crunchy Cinnamon Plantain Strips (p. 242)

day 6

Breakfast: smoothie

Morning snack: Curry Lentil Crackers (p. 259) with Black Bean Lime Salsa (p. 264)

Lunch: Cucumber Pesto Salad (p. 250) with Mango Lime Dressing (p. 254)

Afternoon snack: energy bar

Dinner: Curry Lentil Rice Pizza (p. 239)

After-dinner snack: Arame Seaweed Salad (p. 251)

day 7

Breakfast: Spicy Cocoa Pancakes (p. 214) with raw tahini and fruit

Morning snack: energy bar

Lunch: Zucchini Chip Almond Salad (p. 250) with Ginger Carrot Dressing (p. 254)

Afternoon snack: smoothie

Dinner: Almond Flaxseed Burger (p. 233) with mixed greens and Sweet Pepper Hemp Pesto (p. 267)

After-dinner snack: Zucchini Chips (p. 260)

week 7

day 1

Breakfast: smoothie

Morning snack: Green Tea Ginger Lime Crackers (p. 258) with Black-Eyed Pea Cayenne Salsa (p. 265)

Lunch: Crunchy Cinnamon Plantain and Macadamia Nut Salad (p. 248) with Pomegranate Poppy Seed Dressing (p. 257)

Afternoon snack: energy bar

Dinner: Ginger Lime Squash (p. 241) with Vegetable Crackers (p. 259) and Sunflower Seed Pâté (p. 266)

After-dinner snack: raw vegetables

day 2

Breakfast: smoothie

Morning snack: Lemon Sesame Crisps (p. 260) with fruit

Lunch: Cucumber Pesto Salad (p. 250) with Orange Pumpkin Seed Dressing (p. 255)

Afternoon snack: energy bar

Dinner: Popped Amaranth Rooibos Pizza (p. 239)

After-dinner snack: almonds

day 3

Breakfast: Garlic Oregano Yam Oven Fries (p. 244) with Ketchup (p. 261)

Morning snack: Arame Seaweed Salad (p. 251) with hemp seeds

Lunch: Curry Lentil Rice Pizza (p. 239)

Afternoon snack: energy bar

Dinner: Crunchy Cinnamon Plantain and Macadamia Nut Salad (p. 248) with Caesar Dressing (p. 255)

After-dinner snack: walnuts

day 4

Breakfast: Toasted Apple Cinnamon Cereal (p. 216) with Hemp Milk (p. 268)

Morning snack: energy bar

Lunch: Creamy Carrot Salad (p. 250) with Balsamic Vinaigrette (p. 256)

Afternoon snack: smoothie

Dinner: Adzuki Bean Quinoa Sesame Pizza (p. 237)

After-dinner snack: Zucchini Chips (p. 260)

day 5

Breakfast: smoothie

Morning snack: energy bar

Lunch: Zucchini Chip Almond Salad (p. 250) with Cayenne Dill Tahini Dressing (p. 253)

Afternoon snack: Green Tea Ginger Lime Crackers (p. 258) with Black-Eyed Pea Cayenne Salsa (p. 265)

Dinner: Dinosaur Kale Quinoa Wrap (p. 241) and Sesame Miso Soup (p. 245)

After-dinner snack: Banana Coconut Pie (p. 270)

day 6

Breakfast: Pomegranate Green Tea Pancakes (p. 213) with walnuts and sliced bananas

Morning snack: energy bar

Lunch: Walnut Hemp Burger (p. 233) with mixed greens and Green Tea Miso Gravy (p. 264)

Afternoon snack: smoothie

Dinner: Cucumber Pesto Salad (p. 250) with Tomato Basil Dressing (p. 256)

Morning snack: Vegetable Crackers (p. 259) with Sunflower Seed Pâté (p. 266)

day 7

Breakfast: Banana Ginger Pear Cereal (p. 215) with Chocolate Hemp Milk (p. 268)

Morning snack: energy bar

Lunch: Spicy Black-Eyed Pea Quinoa Pizza (p. 235)

Afternoon snack: raw vegetables and Miso Kelp Guacamole (p. 263)

Dinner: Popped Amaranth Hemp Seed Salad (p. 249) with Cayenne Dill Tahini Dressing (p. 253)

After-dinner snack: Crunchy Cinnamon Plantain Strips (p. 242)

week 8

day 1

Breakfast: smoothie

Morning snack: energy bar

Lunch: Zucchini Chip Almond Salad (p. 250) with Macadamia Dill Dressing (p. 255)

Afternoon snack: Green Tea Ginger Lime Crackers (p. 258) with Black-Eyed Pea Cayenne Salsa (p. 265)

Dinner: Curry Lentil Rice Pizza (p. 239)

After-dinner snack: pistachios

day 2

Breakfast: Lemon Ginger Plantain with Dulse (p. 242) and fruit

Morning snack: green smoothie

Lunch: Sweet Potato Sesame Pizza (p. 238)

Afternoon snack: energy bar

Dinner: Cucumber Pesto Salad (p. 250) with Cayenne Dill Tahini Dressing (p. 253)

After-dinner snack: Sesame Miso Soup (p. 245)

day 3

Breakfast: Toasted Apple Cinnamon Cereal (p. 216) with fruit and Hemp Milk (p. 268)

Morning snack: energy bar

Lunch: Sunflower Seed Beet Pizza (p. 237)

Afternoon snack: Curry Lentil Crackers (p. 259) with Black Bean Lime Salsa (p. 264)

Dinner: Creamy Carrot Salad (p. 250) with Pomegranate Poppy Seed Dressing (p. 257)

After-dinner snack: Creamy Ginger Carrot Soup (p. 245)

day 4

Breakfast: Banana Ginger Pear Cereal (p. 215) with Rooibos Almond Milk (p. 268)

Morning snack: energy bar

Lunch: Cucumber Pesto Salad (p. 250) with Tomato Basil Dressing (p. 256)

Afternoon snack: smoothie

Dinner: Sweet Potato Sesame Pizza (p. 238)

After-dinner snack: Green Soup (p. 246)

day 5

Breakfast: smoothie

Morning snack: Crunchy Cinnamon Plantain Strips (p. 242) with Black-Eyed Pea Cayenne Salsa (p. 265)

Lunch: Popped Amaranth Hemp Seed Salad (p. 249) with Cayenne Dill Tahini Dressing (p. 253)

Afternoon snack: energy bar

Dinner: Walnut Hemp Burger (p. 233) with mixed greens and Mango Chutney (p. 263)

After-dinner snack: raw vegetables and dulse strips

day 6

Breakfast: Wild Rice Yam Pancakes (p. 212) with agave nectar and fruit

Morning snack: energy bar

Lunch: Zucchini Pasta (p. 243) with Spicy Sun-Dried Tomato Marinara Sauce (p. 266) and Creamy Pepper Soup (p. 246)

Afternoon snack: smoothie

Dinner: Cucumber Dill Salad (p. 249) with Macadamia Dill Dressing (p. 255)

After-dinner snack: almonds

day 7

Breakfast: smoothie

Morning snack: energy bar

Lunch: Lemon Crisp Beet Salad (p. 249) with Orange Pumpkin Seed Dressing (p. 255)

Afternoon snack: Zucchini Pasta (p. 243) with Spicy Sun-Dried Tomato Marinara Sauce (p. 266) and Creamy Pepper Soup (p. 246)

Dinner: Dinosaur Kale Quinoa Wrap (p. 241) and Green Tea Ginger Lime Crackers (p. 258) with Black-Eyed Pea Cayenne Salsa (p. 265)

After-dinner snack: Banana Coconut Pie (p. 270)

week 9

day 1

Breakfast: smoothie

Morning snack: energy bar

Lunch: Creamy Carrot Salad (p. 250) with Cayenne Dill Tahini Dressing (p. 253)

Afternoon snack: Crunchy Cinnamon Plantain Strips (p. 242) with Black-Eyed Pea Cayenne Salsa (p. 265)

Dinner: Zucchini Pasta (p. 243) with Spicy Sun-Dried Tomato Marinara Sauce (p. 266) and Creamy Pepper Soup (p. 246)

After-dinner snack: Banana Coconut Pie (p. 270)

day 2

Breakfast: smoothie

Morning snack: energy bar

Lunch: Cucumber Pesto Salad (p. 250) with Tomato Basil Dressing (p. 256)

Afternoon snack: Arame Seaweed Salad (p. 251)

Dinner: Creamy Ginger Carrot Soup (p. 245) and Curry Lentil Crackers (p. 259) with Black Bean Lime Salsa (p. 264)

After-dinner snack: almonds

day 3

Breakfast: Garlic Oregano Yam Oven Fries (p. 244) with Miso Kelp Guacamole (p. 263)

Morning snack: green smoothie

Lunch: Zucchini Pasta (p. 243) with Spicy Sun-Dried Tomato Marinara Sauce (p. 266) and Creamy Pepper Soup (p. 246)

Afternoon snack: energy bar

Dinner: Creamy Carrot Salad (p. 250) with Cayenne Dill Tahini Dressing (p. 253)

After-dinner snack: Zucchini Chips (p. 260)

day 4

Breakfast: Toasted Apple Cinnamon Cereal (p. 216) with fruit and Hemp Milk (p. 268)

Morning snack: energy bar

Lunch: Popped Amaranth Rooibos Pizza (p. 239)

Afternoon snack: smoothie

Dinner: Crunchy Cinnamon Plantain and Macadamia Nut Salad (p. 248) with Tomato Basil Dressing (p. 256)

After-dinner snack: Vegetable Crackers (p. 259) with Sunflower Seed Pâté (p. 266)

day 5

Breakfast: Blueberry Pancakes (p. 213) with agave nectar and fruit

Morning snack: energy bar

Lunch: Cucumber Pesto Salad (p. 250) with Tomato Basil Dressing (p. 256)

Afternoon snack: smoothie

Dinner: Pecan Sunflower Burger (p. 233) with mixed greens and Ginger Carrot Dressing (p. 254) blended with black beans

After-dinner snack: raw vegetables

day 6

Breakfast: smoothie

Morning snack: Crunchy Cinnamon Plantain Strips (p. 242) with Black-Eyed Pea Cayenne Salsa (p. 265)

Lunch: Popped Amaranth Hemp Seed Salad (p. 249) with Cayenne Dill Tahini Dressing (p. 253)

Afternoon snack: energy bar

Dinner: Zucchini Pasta (p. 243) with Macadamia Dill Dressing (p. 255) and Creamy Pepper Soup (p. 246)

After-dinner snack: Arame Seaweed Salad (p. 251)

day 7

Breakfast: Banana Ginger Pear Cereal (p. 215) with Rooibos Almond Milk (p. 268)

Morning snack: energy bar

Lunch: Cucumber Pesto Salad (p. 250) with Balsamic Vinaigrette (p. 256)

Afternoon snack: smoothie

Dinner: Sweet Potato Sesame Pizza (p. 238)

After-dinner snack: Zucchini Chips (p. 260) with Caesar Dressing (p. 255) blended with sunflower seeds

week 10

day 1

Breakfast: Toasted Apple Cinnamon Cereal (p. 216) with fruit and Hemp Milk (p. 268)

Morning snack: energy bar

Lunch: Sunflower Seed Beet Pizza (p. 237)

Afternoon snack: Crunchy Cinnamon Plantain Strips (p. 242) with Black-Eyed Pea Cayenne Salsa (p. 265)

Dinner: Zucchini Chip Almond Salad (p. 250) with Pomegranate Poppy Seed Dressing (p. 257)

After-dinner snack: Vegetable Crackers (p. 259) with Sunflower Seed Pâté (p. 266)

day 2

Breakfast: smoothie

Morning snack: Lemon Rooibos Crackers (p. 258) with Pineapple Salsa (p. 265)

Lunch: Crunchy Cinnamon Plantain and Macadamia Nut Salad (p. 248) with Tomato Basil Dressing (p. 256)

Afternoon snack: energy bar

Dinner: Almond Flaxseed Burger (p. 233) with mixed greens and Black-Eyed Pea Cayenne Salsa (p. 265)

After-dinner snack: Arame Seaweed Salad (p. 251)

day 3

Breakfast: Spicy Cocoa Pancakes (p. 214) with agave nectar and fruit

Morning snack: energy bar

Lunch: Avocado Cayenne Salad (p. 248) with Cucumber Dill Dressing (p. 256)

Afternoon snack: smoothie

Dinner: Almond Flaxseed Burger (p. 233) with mixed greens and Tomato Basil Dressing (p. 256) blended with black beans

After-dinner snack: Zucchini Chips (p. 260)

day 4

Breakfast: Garlic Oregano Yam Oven Fries (p. 244) with Macadamia Dill Dressing (p. 255)

Morning snack: green smoothie

Lunch: Spicy Black-Eyed Pea Quinoa Pizza (p. 235)

Afternoon snack: energy bar

Dinner: Crunchy Cinnamon Plantain and Macadamia Nut Salad (p. 248) with Tomato Basil Dressing (p. 256)

After-dinner snack: Curry Lentil Crackers (p. 259)

day 5

Breakfast: smoothie

Morning snack: energy bar

Lunch: Popped Amaranth Hemp Seed Salad (p. 249) with Orange Pumpkin Seed Dressing (p. 255)

Afternoon snack: honeydew melon

Dinner: Dinosaur Kale Quinoa Wrap (p. 241) and Creamy Pepper Soup (p. 246)

After-dinner snack: raw vegetables

day 6

Breakfast: smoothie

Morning snack: Green Tea Ginger Lime Crackers (p. 258) with Black-Eyed Pea Cayenne Salsa (p. 265)

Lunch: Cucumber Pesto Salad (p. 250) with Ginger Carrot Dressing (p. 254)

Afternoon snack: energy bar

Dinner: Chickpea Curry Pizza (p. 236)

After-dinner snack: fruit

day 7

Breakfast: Toasted Apple Cinnamon Cereal (p. 216) with Hemp Milk (p. 268)

Morning snack: energy bar

Lunch: Lemon Crisp Beet Salad (p. 249) with Tomato Basil Dressing (p. 256)

Afternoon snack: smoothie

Dinner: Curry Lentil Rice Pizza (p. 239)

After-dinner snack: Vegetable Crackers (p. 259) with Caesar Dressing (p. 255) blended with black beans

week 11

day 1

Breakfast: Banana Ginger Pear Cereal (p. 215) with Chocolate Hemp Milk (p. 268)

Morning snack: energy bar

Lunch: Ginger Lime Squash (p. 241)

Afternoon snack: smoothie

Dinner: Popped Amaranth Hemp Seed Salad (p. 249) with Creamy Ginger Dressing (p. 254)

After-dinner snack: Vegetable Crackers (p. 259) with Sunflower Seed Pâté (p. 266)

day 2

Breakfast: smoothie

Morning snack: energy bar

Lunch: Zucchini Chip Almond Salad (p. 250) with Tomato Basil Dressing (p. 256)

Afternoon snack: Curry Lentil Crackers (p. 259) with Macadamia Dill Dressing (p. 255)

Dinner: Dinosaur Kale Quinoa Wrap (p. 241) and Creamy Ginger Carrot Soup (p. 245)

After-dinner snack: Banana Coconut Pie (p. 270)

day 3

Breakfast: Buckwheat Pancakes (p. 212) with agave nectar and fruit

Morning snack: energy bar

Lunch: Creamy Carrot Salad (p. 250) with Tomato Basil Dressing (p. 256)

Afternoon snack: smoothie

Dinner: Pecan Sunflower Burger (p. 233) with mixed greens and Pineapple Salsa (p. 265)

After-dinner snack: Crunchy Cinnamon Plantain Strips (p. 242)

day 4

Breakfast: smoothie

Morning snack: watermelon

Lunch: Cucumber Pesto Salad (p. 250) with Mango Lime Dressing (p. 254)

Afternoon snack: energy bar

Dinner: Creamy Pepper Soup (p. 246) and Zucchini Pasta (p. 243) with Caesar Dressing (p. 255) blended with black-eyed peas

After-dinner snack: pistachios

day 5

Breakfast: smoothie

Morning snack: Curry Lentil Crackers (p. 259) with Mango Chutney (p. 263)

Lunch: Cucumber Pesto Salad (p. 250) with Tomato Basil Dressing (p. 256)

Afternoon snack: energy bar

Dinner: Sunflower Seed Beet Pizza (p. 237)

After-dinner snack: raw vegetables with Sunflower Seed Pâté (p. 266)

day 6

Breakfast: Toasted Apple Cinnamon Cereal (p. 216) with fruit and Hemp Milk (p. 268)

Morning snack: energy bar

Lunch: Crunchy Cinnamon Plantain and Macadamia Nut Salad (p. 248) with Tomato Basil Dressing (p. 256)

Afternoon snack: smoothie

Dinner: Chickpea Curry Pizza (p. 236)

After-dinner snack: Arame Seaweed Salad (p. 251)

day 7

Breakfast: Garlic Oregano Yam Oven Fries (p. 244) with Mango Lime Dressing (p. 254)

Morning snack: green smoothie

Lunch: Curry Lentil Rice Pizza (p. 239)

Afternoon snack: energy bar

Dinner: Cucumber Pesto Salad (p. 250) with Tomato Basil Dressing (p. 256)

After-dinner snack: Crunchy Cinnamon Plantain Strips (p. 242)

week 12

day 1

Breakfast: smoothie

Morning snack: energy bar

Lunch: Creamy Carrot Salad (p. 250) with Cucumber Dill Dressing (p. 256)

Afternoon snack: honeydew melon

Dinner: Dinosaur Kale Quinoa Wrap (p. 241) and Sesame Miso Soup (p. 245)

After-dinner snack: Banana Coconut Pie (p. 270)

day 2

Breakfast: smoothie

Morning snack: energy bar

Lunch: Pecan Sunflower Burger (p. 233) with mixed greens and Tomato Basil Dressing (p. 256) blended with black beans

Afternoon snack: raw vegetables with Caesar Dressing (p. 255)

Dinner: Creamy Carrot Salad (p. 250) with Cayenne Dill Tahini Dressing (p. 253)

After-dinner snack: pumpkin seeds

day 3

Breakfast: Banana Ginger Pear Cereal (p. 215) with Rooibos Almond Milk (p. 268)

Morning snack: energy bar

Lunch: Sunflower Seed Beet Pizza (p. 237)

Afternoon snack: raw vegetables with Pomegranate Poppy Seed Dressing (p. 257)

Dinner: Avocado Cayenne Salad (p. 248) with Balsamic Vinaigrette (p. 256)

After-dinner snack: Sesame Miso Soup (p. 245)

day 4

Breakfast: Pomegranate Green Tea Pancakes (p. 213) with raw tahini and fruit

Morning snack: green smoothie

Lunch: Chickpea Curry Pizza (p. 236)

Afternoon snack: energy bar

Dinner: Cucumber Pesto Salad (p. 250) with Ginger Carrot Dressing (p. 254)

After-dinner snack: raw vegetables with Macadamia Dill Dressing (p. 255)

day 5

Breakfast: smoothie

Morning snack: fruit

Lunch: Crunchy Cinnamon Plantain and Macadamia Nut Salad (p. 248) with Cayenne Dill Tahini Dressing (p. 253)

Afternoon snack: energy bar

Dinner: Spicy Black-Eyed Pea Quinoa Pizza (p. 235)

After-dinner snack: pumpkin seeds

day 6

Breakfast: Toasted Apple Cinnamon Cereal (p. 216) with Hemp Milk (p. 268) and fruit

Morning snack: energy bar

Lunch: Cucumber Pesto Salad (p. 250) with Tomato Basil Dressing (p. 256)

Afternoon snack: smoothie

Dinner: Popped Amaranth Rooibos Pizza (p. 239)

After-dinner snack: Zucchini Chips (p. 260) with Ginger Carrot Dressing (p. 254)

day 7

Breakfast: Spicy Cocoa Pancakes (p. 214) with raw almond butter and fruit

Morning snack: energy bar

Lunch: Crunchy Cinnamon Plantain and Macadamia Nut Salad (p. 248) with Balsamic Vinaigrette (p. 256)

Afternoon snack: smoothie

Dinner: Pecan Sunflower Burger (p. 233) with mixed greens and Mango Lime Dressing (p. 254)

After-dinner snack: raw vegetables

seven

recipes for the thrive diet

my recipe philosophy

I try to use as few ingredients as possible in each recipe. I appreciate simple, clean, well-balanced flavor. Each ingredient in my recipes serves a purpose. The ingredients are combined in such a way that you will begin to notice and appreciate the subtleties that each offers without being bombarded with an overabundance of flavors. Apart from simply tasting cleaner, Thrive Diet foods will help the body become aware of, and value, truly fresh, tasty food. In doing so, your sensory system will naturally gravitate toward these foods and away from over-flavored ones. The reason refined foods are so rich in flavor is simply because flavor is added—lots of it. Once naturally flavorful whole food is stripped of its nutrition, it is virtually tasteless. So, in an attempt to compensate for the loss of natural flavor, processed foods are flavored—usually greatly over-flavored. As with sensory stimulation in our society, our flavor-sensing ability could stand an overhaul. Like stimulation, the best way to reintroduce simple flavor is to recalibrate. Using fewer ingredients in a recipe will do that. As a result, the body will be less inclined to consume processed foods, helping it break cravings.

Fewer ingredients also mean a quicker, easier-to-prepare meal or snack, which I certainly welcome. I like to be able to prepare complete balanced meals and nourishing snacks within a few minutes. With some planning, none of these recipes, even the main courses, will take much longer than 30 minutes to prepare.

You may notice that several healthy fruits and vegetables are not included in the recipes; this is because I structured the meal plan on foods that are commonly available. If you have access to more exotic fruits and vegetables that fit the premise of the Thrive Diet, by all means incorporate them into the recipes and meal plan.

Thrive Diet recipes don't state calorie, carbohydrate, protein, or fat values. This information is not important in the Thrive Diet: Assessing food value based on calories, carbohydrate, protein, and fat is not a reliable measure of nutrition. Simply by adhering to the Thrive Diet principles, the body will be supplied with all the nutrition it needs—all the bases will be covered without having to aim for certain quantities of macronutrients. One of the appeals of the Thrive Diet is its simplicity, which allows the diet to become more of a way of life than a program to be followed.

As with variations between wines, there will be variations in natural food dishes, depending on each crop of the ingredients: Crops vary from yield to yield, affecting the flavor and texture of the food, and also the moisture levels. Because of this, the Thrive Diet recipes may turn out slightly differently each time you prepare them.

herbs

For recipes calling for herbs, the measures are for the dried form unless they must be fresh. In some recipes, either can be used, and I've noted this. Fresh herbs are always the best choice, but I realize that they are not always available. If space, light, and time allow, growing your own herbs is a practical way to ensure you always have the premium fresh form available. Along with taste, nutritional value is superior in the fresh plant. Whole plants are available in most garden stores for under a dollar each. If you put them in a spacious container, ensure that they get plenty of natural light, and water them a few times a week, they will provide a worthwhile bounty. Basic herbs that are low maintenance and easy to grow include:

Basil
Chives
Cilantro
Coriander
Dill
Mint
Oregano
Parsley
Thyme

soaking and sprouting

Soaking nuts and seeds is an easy way to improve their digestibility and increase their nutritional value. Soaking them for as little as four hours can yield a significant benefit. Each week or so, I put a variety of raw nuts and seeds into separate bowls and then cover them with purified water and leave them to sit overnight on the counter. I do this in the evening, then, when I get up in the morning, I drain the water, rinse the nuts and seeds with fresh water (being sure to rinse well, to wash off the digestive inhibitors that have leached into the water, thus improving bioavailability), and store them in the refrigerator. This way they are on hand when making meals.

It takes me really only about 10 minutes a week to soak the nuts, so the time commitment is small; it simply takes forethought. Almonds, pumpkin seeds, and sesame seeds are the ones I most often soak. These seeds won't sprout, but they will benefit nutritionally from being soaked.

Soaked raw nuts are always better from a nutritional standpoint than their unsoaked counterparts. However, with the exception of those called for in the nut milks and my Zucchini Chip Almond Salad (recipe on page 250) the nuts and seeds for the Thrive Diet recipes do not need to be soaked first—they can be used in the recipes as they are.

Sprouting grains and legumes is a lengthier process than soaking, but not really that much more of a time commitment on your part. For the recipes in this book, you may choose to use canned, precooked, ready-to-eat legumes. This is the most convenient way to get your legumes for recipes. A wide variety of lentils and other legumes, including chickpeas and adzuki beans, are available in this form and can be found in supermarkets and many convenience stores. Look for legumes that are packed without the use of preservatives.

Or you may choose to cook the legumes yourself. This is less expensive than buying canned legumes, but be aware that cooking times range from 20 minutes for lentils all the way up to three hours for chickpeas. I would rather gain the greatest nutrition by simply planning ahead, and sprouting my grains and legumes.

Buying sprouts are an option—many types can be bought in supermarkets and most health food stores with cold storage. However, store-bought sprouts have been known to harbor bacteria. If your immune system is low and you are in a compromised state of health, you will likely want to avoid this risk. I highly recommend buying the raw grains and legumes and sprouting them yourself. It takes a bit of planning, but the nutritional gains reaped are worth it.

The sprout occupies a transitional phase in the plant life cycle. Having yet to form roots, the sprout, a new growth from the germinating seed, cannot feed itself and so must rely on the nutrients contained within the seed. Once activated by moisture, enzymes begin to utilize nutrients supplied in the seed as a rapid growth fuel. The plant equivalent of mother's milk, densely packed nutrients in the seed quickly convert the sprout into a plant with leaves.

The sprout has much to offer. Throughout the sprout's rapid growth phase, digestive enzyme inhibitors are expelled; proteins are converted to amino acids, and fats to essential fatty acids; and a form of pre-digestion occurs, making for a very efficient food. Power-packed with vitamins, minerals, chlorophyll, and enzymes, sprouting greatly enhances the efficiency and nutrient value of the seed. Sprouts, because of their high pH level, will also help alkalize the body. Most grains, legumes, nuts, and seeds can be sprouted. (Some seeds, including sunflower seeds, will develop shoots. Sesame seeds and pumpkin seeds will not sprout but will benefit from being soaked.) Quinoa and buckwheat are especially good for sprouting, as sprouting unleashes their full array of nutrients.

Should you choose to try sprouting, you will likely find that sprouting quickly becomes a part of your daily routine. It's very easy to do and has an extra bonus of low cost. Canned legumes are not expensive, but sprouting dried seeds, grains, and legumes is dirt cheap.

Although any uncooked legume, nut, grain, and seed will benefit from being soaked or sprouted, these ones work particular well and are easy to incorporate into several of the Thrive Diet recipes:

soaking	**sprouting**
Almonds	Amaranth
Macadamia nuts	Buckwheat
Pumpkin seeds	Beans, all kinds
Sesame seeds	Chickpeas
Oats	Lentils, all kinds (can also be just soaked to save time)
Wild rice	Quinoa
	Sunflower seeds

how to sprout

Sprouting kits are available in most health food stores; these make sprouting easier, but they are not essential. All you need is a jar, cheesecloth, and an elastic band.

Rinse well whatever you intend to sprout and pour it into a glass jar, to about the one-quarter mark. Fill the jar at least three-quarters full with water. Let it sit overnight at room temperature. Pour out the water and rinse the legumes, grains, nuts, or seeds with fresh water. Put them back in the jar and put the cheesecloth over the top, holding it down with the elastic band. Briefly turn the jar upside down to let the water drain out. Within about 24 hours, the sprouts will begin to appear. Make sure the sprouts stay moist so that they will sprout fully; do this by pouring water into the jar and then turning it upside down to drain.

The sprouting time depends on the type of sprouts; two days is typical. Rinse the sprouts in fresh water. This will wash off the digestive inhibitors that have leached into the water, thus improving bioavailability. Store the sprouts in a clean, uncovered container in the refrigerator; they will keep for up to one week.

variations

seeds and flour

To keep the recipes interesting, I've included variations for several. As well, since none of the recipes uses glutinous flour, flours can be easily substituted for one another in those recipes calling for flour. Seed flours, including hemp, flaxseed, and sesame seed flours, rather than grain flours, are the best choice (you'll notice that seeds are lower to the base of the Thrive Diet pyramid [see page 40] than grains).

Another way to enhance nutrient value and infuse recipes with an alkaline source of protein, essential fatty acids, and greens is to substitute my Vega Whole Food Smoothie Infusion formula, available in most health food and grocery stores, for ground seeds or flour. This formula can be used in place of non-glutinous flour at a 1:1 ratio.

You will notice that some recipes call for hemp protein; this can be replaced with hemp flour if you prefer. Hemp protein is a bit more expensive because it has been milled further, removing more of the starch. Hemp flour is about 35 percent protein, whereas hemp protein is about 50 percent protein.

carob

Carob pods, which grow up to one foot in length, are the fruit of the carob tree and are quite high in trace minerals. Raw carob powder is relatively easy to find in stores, but its flavor is quite mild. A good raw alternative is cacao (often called raw chocolate), but it is more difficult to find. Also, it contains a bit of caffeine. For these reasons, I tend to use roasted carob powder for chocolate flavor.

oil

I use hemp oil as the base for salad dressings, sauces, and many other recipes that do not require cooking at high heat. This is because hemp offers exceptional flavor and nutrition, as you have read. Using only hemp oil as your primary oil source is a good way to go; however, a blend of about 80 percent hemp oil, 10 percent flaxseed oil, and 10 percent pumpkin seed oil is an optimal balance of essential fatty acids. I've written in detail about the health benefits of each of these seed oils on pages 143–145. This combination can be used in place of just hemp oil for variety and for an improved essential fatty acid profile, though its use is not necessary to reap the benefits of the Thrive Diet. You'll find the recipe for the EFA Oil Blend on page 210.

If you want to step it up another notch, add small amounts of berry seed oils to the blend. These are packed with antioxidants in a highly concentrated form. Raspberry, cranberry, and pomegranate seed oils are among the best. They can be hard to find in stores and are expensive, but they will deliver an extra dimension to a high-quality oil blend. A mixture containing all these oils is the ultimate essential fatty acid and antioxidant combination. However, it is not necessary to use these oils to achieve results on the Thrive Diet. Or, you might choose to use my Vega Antioxidant EFA Oil Blend formula, available in most health food and grocery stores (see Resources).

juice

For the recipes that require juices, I usually juice the fruit myself instead of using store-bought juice. Lemons, limes, and oranges are easy to juice simply by squeezing (warming to room temperature for about 10 minutes first will yield the most juice). Home-squeezed juices are, of course, unpasteurized and therefore retain more goodness and taste better than many commercial versions. There are, however, some good store-bought products. Just Juice brand is a good one: it's pure juice, and because it's not from concentrate, it offers a higher level of nutrition (see Resources).

salt

You will notice that I usually don't give a specific measure for salt in my recipes. This is because sodium requirements and tastes vary quite widely. Simply add sea salt to taste. Since the Thrive Diet does not include any processed or manufactured foods, it is a low-sodium diet, and adding a bit of sea salt to certain recipes will not have a negative impact on your health. Sea salt is generally of greater value than its mined counterpart: It contains more trace minerals and is less processed.

Alternatively, you could use dulse flakes as a healthy substitute for sea salt. Grind the flakes into a powder in a coffee grinder and keeping them on hand to use in place of salt. You will need to use about twice as much dulse powder as you would salt to achieve the same saltiness. Dried dulse flakes are available at most health food stores. Kelp flakes are another good option, though they have more of an ocean taste and so are suitable in fewer recipes.

recipes

variations

For extra nutritional value, hemp protein and ground flaxseeds can be substituted in all recipes, including baked ones, for Vega Whole Food Smoothie Infusion on a 1:1 ratio. Vega Whole Food Health Optimizer can also be used to replace hemp and ground flaxseeds on a 1:1 ratio, but only for non-heated recipes, since heat will destroy the value of its probiotics.

Thrive Diet basics

These recipes are designed to be made ahead of time and kept on-hand for use in other Thrive Diet recipes.

Popped Amaranth

Light and fluffy, popped amaranth is a nice substitute for heavier flours in pancakes; it also adds texture to energy bars and crunch to salads. Keep refrigerated for up to 2 weeks (because of its natural oils, it needs to be refrigerated).

Use a hot air popcorn popper and pop amaranth as you would corn.

Amaranth can also be popped in a frying pan:

Heat a small amount of coconut oil, just enough to cover the bottom of the pan, over medium heat. Add a small amount of amaranth, just enough to cover the bottom of the pan. As it pops, remove it from the pan with a spatula and add more grains for popping.

EFA Oil Blend

raw

- 8 parts hemp oil
- 1 part flaxseed oil
- 1 part pumpkin seed oil

Combine all ingredients.

* To further boost nutritional value and antioxidant level, this blend can be substituted in all recipes for Vega Antioxidant EFA Oil Blend.

Keep refrigerated.

Curry Powder

Although some store-bought curry powders are quite good, this mixture guarantees a pungent, authentic flavor. Make up a batch to have on hand as a seasoning for various dishes.

- 2 tbsp coriander
- 2 tbsp cumin
- 2 tsp cardamom
- 1 1/2 tsp cinnamon
- 1 tsp black pepper
- 1 tsp cloves
- 1 tsp nutmeg
- 1 tsp turmeric
- 1/2 tsp cayenne pepper

Combine all ingredients; store in an air-tight jar.

Variation: Add 2 tsp of lime zest for tang.

Makes 3/4 cup.

Nutritional Yeast and Sesame Seed Topping

Since nutritional yeast melts, this topping adds a creamy texture to any warm food. Its flavor closely resembles that of mild cheddar cheese. It can be used in place of Parmesan cheese in any recipe. The high level of B vitamins in the nutritional yeast and the calcium from the sesame seeds make this topping a nutrient-packed boost.

I make a couple of cups of this topping at a time and put it in a cheese shaker so that it's always handy. Keep in the refrigerator to prevent the oil in the sesame seeds from going rancid.

1 part nutritional yeast flakes
1 part unhulled sesame seeds

Grind nutritional yeast flakes and sesame seeds together in a coffee grinder.

pancakes

These pancakes are much more filling than the traditional fluffy variety made with refined carbohydrate. Since their base ingredients are a combination of flaxseed, hemp, and pseudograins, they are packed with nourishment.

Following the Thrive Diet principle of cooking only at low heat, and since these pancakes contain essential fatty acids that are destroyed at high heat, they are cooked at a low temperature.

I've included baking powder and baking soda in some of these recipes to make the pancakes a bit fluffier. I usually omit both since I prefer denser pancakes, and if you do too, feel free to omit them also.

Agave nectar is a good alternative to maple syrup as a pancake topping.

Pancake Procedure Follow this procedure for all the pancake recipes, unless otherwise specified:

In a food processor, process all ingredients until smooth.

Lightly oil a pan with coconut oil and heat over medium heat. Pour in pancake batter to desired pancake size and cook for about 5 minutes or until bubbles begin to appear. Flip and allow to cook for another 5 minutes.

Buckwheat Pancakes

Lightly flavored with cinnamon and nutmeg, these pancakes taste more like traditional pancakes than the other Thrive Diet pancakes.

1 cup buckwheat flour
1/4 cup ground flaxseed
1/4 cup hemp flour
2 tsp baking powder
1 tsp cinnamon
1/2 tsp nutmeg
1 banana
2 cups water
1/2 cup barley flakes (or buckwheat, sprouted or cooked)

In a bowl, mix buckwheat flour, flaxseed, hemp flour, baking powder, cinnamon, and nutmeg. In a food processor, process the banana and water while slowly adding the dry ingredients, until mixture is smooth. Stir in the barley flakes with a spoon or spatula.

Cook as directed above.

Makes 2 large servings.

Wild Rice Yam Pancakes

This is a heartier mixture than traditional pancakes, one that will give you a sense of fullness for several hours.

2 cups water
1 cup cooked or sprouted quinoa

cont.

1 cup mashed cooked yam
1/2 cup sprouted or cooked wild rice
1/4 cup ground flaxseed
1/4 cup ground sesame seeds
2 tsp baking powder
1/2 tsp black pepper

Makes 2 large servings.

Blueberry Pancakes

These are similar to traditional blueberry pancakes but with usable nutrition.

2 fresh or soaked dried dates
1 cup blueberries
1 cup Hemp Milk (p. 268)
3/4 cup water
1/2 cup buckwheat flour
1/2 cup sprouted or cooked quinoa
1 tsp baking powder
1 tsp baking soda
Sea salt to taste

Makes 2 large servings.

Pomegranate Green Tea Pancakes

A flavorful mixture containing antioxidants, this recipe will supply the nutrients needed for a busy day.

2 fresh or soaked dried dates
1 cup pomegranate seeds (the amount from 1 pomegranate)
1 cup Hemp Milk (p. 268)
3/4 cup water
1/2 cup Popped Amaranth (p. 209)
1/2 cup rice flour
1 tbsp finely ground green tea leaves (or 1 tsp matcha powder)
1 tsp baking powder

cont.

1 tsp baking soda
Sea salt to taste

Makes 2 large servings.

Banana Chocolate Pancakes

Designed with kids in mind, these pancakes are popular for weekday breakfasts. Unlike traditional breakfasts that most children eat, these pancakes are packed with high-quality protein, essential fatty acids, and naturally occurring vitamins and minerals.

2 bananas
2 fresh or soaked dried dates
1 cup Popped Amaranth (p. 209)
1 cup Chocolate Hemp Milk (p. 268)
1 cup water
1/2 cup buckwheat flour
1/4 cup ground flaxseed
1/4 cup hemp flour
1/4 cup roasted carob powder
1/4 cup unsweetened carob chips
Sea salt to taste

Makes 2 large servings.

Spicy Cocoa Pancakes

The cayenne gives these nutrient-packed pancakes a bit of heat and encourages blood flow.

2 bananas
1 date
1/2 cup buckwheat flour
1/2 cup sprouted or cooked quinoa
1/4 cup roasted carob powder
1/4 cup ground flaxseed
1/4 cup hemp flour

cont.

1/2 tsp cayenne pepper

Sea salt to taste

Makes 2 large servings.

cereals

Cereals are one of the most popular breakfast foods in North America, and for good reason. They are tasty, fast and easy to prepare, and come in a variety of flavors and textures. The problem is that most commercial versions don't offer nutrient density and certainly don't provide balanced nutrition. This usually means you're hungry not long after eating a bowl of cereal.

Thrive Diet cereals consist of fiber, protein, and essential fatty acids, along with many whole-food source vitamins and minerals. This gives them staying power.

Banana Ginger Pear Cereal

raw option

On the mornings that I have slightly more time, I'll often make Banana Ginger Pear Cereal as a change from my usual smoothie. It is still quick to prepare and makes for a balanced meal. Since most commercial cereals are based on refined grains and laden with sugar, this is a far superior option. To make this cereal even more nutritious, top with an energy bar (recipes begin on page 226), cut into small pieces.

1 banana

1 pear

1 date

1/4 cup almonds

1 tbsp ground flaxseed

1 tbsp hemp flour

1/2 tbsp roasted carob powder (or cacao nibs to make cereal 100% raw)

1/2 tbsp grated fresh ginger

cont.

Slice banana into bite-size pieces. Core pear and slice into bite-size pieces. Pit and cut date into small pieces. Chop almonds into desired size. Combine all ingredients in a bowl; stir. Top with Hemp Milk (p. 268) or Rooibos Almond Milk (p. 268).

Variation: Add 1/2 cup sprouted buckwheat or quinoa.

Makes 1 large serving.

Toasted Apple Cinnamon Cereal

This is an excellent cereal in terms of nutritional balance. Unlike many commercial cereals, this one has lots of fiber, complete protein, essential fatty acids, and calcium.

1/2 apple, diced
1 cup oats (or cooked or sprouted quinoa to make cereal gluten-free)
1/2 cup diced almonds
1/2 cup ground flaxseed
1/2 cup hemp flour
1/2 cup unhulled sesame seeds
1/2 cup sunflower seeds
1 1/2 tsp cinnamon
1/4 tsp nutmeg
1/4 tsp ground stevia leaf
1/4 tsp sea salt
1/4 cup hemp oil or EFA Oil Blend (p. 210)
1/4 cup molasses
2 tbsp apple juice

Preheat oven to 250°F.

Combine apple, oats, almonds, ground flaxseed, hemp flour, sesame seeds, sunflower seeds, cinnamon, nutmeg, stevia, and sea salt. Blend together hemp oil, molasses, and apple juice. Combine liquid and dry ingredients, mixing well.

Spread on a baking tray lightly oiled with coconut oil. Bake for 1 hour. Let cool, then break into pieces.

Keep refrigerated for up to 2 weeks.

Makes 4 cups or about 5 servings.

smoothies

the basics

Ideally, a smoothie will contain all the nutrients of a complete meal. The protein should be from an easily digestible source, otherwise, one of the health-promoting benefits a smoothie offers—ease of digestibility—will be reduced. The protein is best obtained from whole food that has a high pH, and at least a portion of it should be derived from a raw source, such as hemp. Raw hemp protein is packed with live enzymes that improve digestion and absorption, and provides a high amount of complete protein. I always use hemp as my primary protein source when making a smoothie. I also include ground flaxseed, for its omega-3 and omega-6 fatty acids, lignans, and fiber. With these basics, you can make a nutritious, tasty smoothie by simply adding fresh or frozen fruit. The fruit provides a healthy source of carbohydrate, antioxidants, and enzymes. Vega Whole Food Smoothie Infusion may be substituted for hemp protein or flaxseed on a 1:1 ratio.

the next level

To take these smoothie recipes or your own concoctions to the next level in terms of nutrition, add next-level ingredients. These foods will infuse smoothies with nutrient-rich whole foods. Although none is essential to achieve the results of the Thrive Diet, by including them, the body will realize the benefits more quickly.

Instead of making the smoothie recipes in this book, you may choose to simply use Vega Whole Food Health Optimizer, a convenient powder formula that I developed. This ready-made smoothie mix embodies the principles of the Thrive Diet and provides all the next-level ingredients in addition to the smoothie basics. It is available in most health food stores and supermarkets.

A Balanced Amino Acid Profile: Rice and Pea Combined with Hemp In an attempt to optimize the nutritional value of my smoothies, I began adding yellow pea and rice protein powder to balance the amino acid profile and improve the quality of protein. When I combined several protein sources, I found that my ability to recover improved dramatically. Improved recovery is an indication that the body has been relieved of stress. I noticed immediate gains in strength and lean muscle retention, even during times of elevated stress. The desire to consume more food dissipated as well, leaving me leaner.

Amino acid levels vary in all protein sources. By synergistically selecting complementary sources and amounts, we can achieve what is known as a flatline profile. The flatline profile of properly combined amino acids is an indicator that all amino acids are being met in substantial quantities and is a broad-spectrum source of protein.

Found predominantly in hemp, edestin is an easily digestible form of protein. Beneficial to the structural integrity of our cells' DNA, edestin more closely resembles human protein than any other in the plant kingdom. The branch-chain amino acids leucine, isoleucine, and valine are also plentiful in hemp protein. Essential for the repair and building of lean muscle tissue, these branch-chain amino acids are also an integral part of maintaining a healthy metabolic rate.

Hemp protein by itself is complete, but there is still room for improvement. Because it is relatively low in the essential amino acid tryptophan, hemp protein is nicely complemented by rice protein. Prominent in rice protein, tryptophan helps the body fabricate serotonin. With more readily available serotonin in the system, mood will be elevated, resulting in fewer sugar and starch cravings.

Relatively hard to find in the plant kingdom, the amino acid lysine is exceptionally high in yellow pea protein. An essential amino acid, lysine is critical in the body's production of enzymes, antibodies, and hormones. The body's ability to maintain correct nitrogen balance and absorb calcium is also reliant on the presence of lysine in the diet. During times of augmented stress, eating lysine-rich foods will help maintain lean muscle tissue.

The combination of hemp, yellow pea, and rice protein is not only complete, it is complementary and synergistic, structured better than any single protein source can ever be. However, because pea protein and rice protein can be difficult to find, the recipes below call simply for hemp protein and ground flaxseed. If you simply follow the 12-Week Meal Plan, you will reap the rewards a variety of properly combined proteins deliver. But if you *are* able to source these proteins, by all means include them in your smoothies. Add 10 grams (4 teaspoons) of pea protein and 5 grams (2 teaspoons) of rice protein along with the hemp protein.

Maca In my Vega Whole Food Health Optimizer formula, I include maca. (I discuss its benefits in detail on page 154.) A root vegetable related to the turnip, maca is an adrenal tonic. Although maca is not an essential part of the Thrive Diet, it is of particular use when feeling depleted, to help speed the rate at which the adrenals can be rebuilt after bouts of high stress. Aside from its myriad nutrients (trace amounts of 31 minerals), maca supplies the body with a non-stimulating form of energy. Maca delivers energy by means of hormonal regulation and adrenal nourishment, not stimulation. As the diet improves, maca's energy-inducing properties become increasingly apparent.

The principles of the Thrive Diet, of course, are ones of nourishment that extend to the adrenals; maca can speed the process at which they regenerate. Including maca in a smoothie is also a sensible way to help rebuild the adrenal glands after the use of a stimulant such as yerba maté during times of production stress. When I have to perform at a particularly high level, whether for a key workout, race, or the completion of a major project, I sometimes drink yerba maté. It works. I get more energy, but at the expense of my adrenals. Without fail, during these times and immediately afterward, I make sure to have a daily dose of maca to speed the regeneration process. Several of my exercise-specific recipes (pages 122–129) have the option of including yerba maté; if you do, take maca afterward.

Add: 2.5 grams (1 tsp) of gelatinized maca.

Chlorella Chlorella is another highly beneficial food that I add to my smoothies. (I discuss chlorella in detail on page 150.) A fresh water algae, chlorella possesses many detoxifying properties that can help speed the rate at which the body rids itself of toxins. The Thrive Diet is one of cleansing; consuming chlorella daily will speed the rate at which that takes place. Toxins are constantly being taken into our bodies with the air we breathe and the food we eat, and the more toxins within our body, the more stress placed on our system as a whole.

Add: 2.5 grams (1 tsp) chlorella.

Probiotics Probiotics are the "good" bacteria in our intestines (see the Glossary for a more detailed description). As mentioned in Chapter 1, if nutrient-rich whole foods are not primary in your diet, cravings and overeating will develop. If they persist even once you adhere to a nutrient-rich diet, the problem might be absorption. Once food has been digested in the stomach, it passes into the intestine, where the vitamins and minerals are absorbed for utilization. If good bacteria are not prevalent in the intestine, the absorption process will be hindered. Not being able to utilize vitamin-rich foods is just as bad as not consuming them in the first place.

Too often, when we get a bacterial infection, we are given antibiotics to kill it. The problem with this is that antibiotics also kill good bacteria. Increasingly, antibiotics aren't working as effectively as they have in the past, as many bacteria have developed a resistance to them. Prevention is the way to go. By consuming probiotics on a weekly basis, your chance of infection—and therefore the need for antibiotics—is greatly reduced. Consistent probiotic use has shown to dramatically improve immune function. You may choose to add non-dairy probiotics, such as store-bought soil-based ones, which come in both capsule and powder form, to your smoothies. Other sources include brown rice miso paste, which you'll find in a few of the Thrive Diet recipes. It's not necessary to consume probiotics daily; a few times a week is plenty if you are already eating a healthy diet that does not combat probiotics.

Add: 1/4 tsp soil probiotics.

Extra Essential Fatty Acids Even though the ground flaxseed and hemp protein called for in the smoothie recipes below supply a solid amount of essential fatty acids, you may choose to add oil as well. As with the salad dressings, hemp is a good option, but a blend of several oils will ensure diversity among nutrients. I'll often mix hemp oil with flaxseed and pumpkin seed oils. You'll find the recipe for this blend, which I call EFA Oil Blend, on page 210.

variation

One of the best things about smoothies other than their nutritional density and convenience is the variety that they offer. I've provided a few of my favorite recipes below, but feel free to get creative and use other fruits and vegetables, in any combination. For times when you feel especially hungry, add sprouted buckwheat or other pseudograin. When you start with base ingredients that deliver high-quality protein and essential fatty acids, such as hemp and flaxseed, you can't go wrong no matter what fruits and vegetables you add.

I use fresh fruit when it's in season. Frozen fruit is a good alternative—look for frozen fruit that does not contain any preservatives; it is pretty much on par with its fresh counterpart. I usually peel and freeze bananas ahead of time so that I have a handy supply at all times. Adding them frozen to the smoothie is like adding a form of ice, and it helps blend all the ingredients together for a smooth, thick consistency. You can also substitute ice cubes for some of the water. Using frozen fruit and ice cubes makes the smoothies thicker, which seems to ward off hunger even longer. For extra flavor and electrolytes, substitute coconut water for water in any of the smoothie recipes.

Smoothie Procedure For all the smoothie recipes, simply blend all the ingredients together in a blender.

* To further increase nutritional value of all smoothies, substitute hemp protein and ground flaxseeds with Vega Whole Food Smoothie Infusion or Vega Whole Food Health Optimizer on a 1:1 ratio.

All smoothies can be kept refrigerated for up to 3 days, though they're best when fresh.

Ginger Pear Smoothie *(inflammation reducer)*

raw

This is a refreshingly crisp smoothie. It's not too sweet, although the riper the pear, the sweeter it will be. If you want it sweeter, add one or two fresh or soaked dried dates.

- 1 banana
- 1/2 pear, cored
- 2 cups cold water (or 1 1/2 cups water plus 1 cup ice)
- 1 tbsp ground flaxseed
- 1 tbsp hemp protein
- 1 tbsp grated ginger

Makes about 3 cups, or 2 servings.

Chocolate Almond Smoothie *(antioxidant-rich)*

raw option

This is a satisfying smoothie that will keep the hunger away for hours.

- 1 banana
- 2 fresh or soaked dried dates
- 2 cups cold water (or 1 1/2 cups water plus 1 cup ice)
- 1/4 cup almonds (or 2 tbsp raw almond butter)
- 1 tbsp ground flaxseed
- 1 tbsp hemp protein
- 1 tbsp roasted carob powder (or cacao nibs to make smoothie 100% raw)

Makes about 3 1/2 cups, or 2 large servings.

Tropical Pineapple Mango Smoothie *(quick, non-stimulating energy)*

raw

Papain in papaya and bromelain in pineapple are active digestive enzymes that will help speed digestion. This is a good smoothie when you're on the go or after a hard workout, when the body is fatigued, since it is digested even more quickly than the others.

- 1 banana
- 2 fresh or soaked dried dates
- 2 cups cold water (or 1 1/2 cups water plus 1 cup ice)
- 1/2 medium papaya

cont.

1/2 cup pineapple
1 tbsp ground flaxseed
1 tbsp hemp protein
1 tbsp coconut oil

Makes about 3 1/2 cups, or 2 large servings.

Blueberry Rooibos Antioxidant Smoothie *(antioxidant-rich)*

The many antioxidants in this smoothie will mop up cell-damaging free-radicals produced by stress.

1 banana
2 cups cold water (or 1 1/2 cups water plus 1 cup ice)
1/2 cup blueberries
1 tbsp ground flaxseed
1 tbsp hemp protein
1 tbsp agave nectar
1 tbsp hemp oil or EFA Oil Blend (p. 210)
2 tsp ground rooibos

Makes about 3 1/2 cups, or 2 large servings.

Blood Builder Smoothie *(iron-rich)*

raw

The vitamin C–rich orange in this smoothie will help the body absorb the iron of the pumpkin seeds.

1 banana
1 orange
2 cups cold water (or 1 1/2 cups water plus 1 cup ice)
2 tbsp pumpkin seeds
1 tbsp ground flaxseed
1 tbsp hemp protein
1 tbsp agave nectar
1 tbsp hemp oil or EFA Oil Blend (p. 210)
1/4 tsp cloves

Makes about 3 1/2 cups, or 2 large servings.

Mango Lime Hot Pepper Smoothie *(immune booster)*

This smoothie will help get the blood flowing more quickly, creating a feeling of warmth. Its high level of vitamin A and vitamin C help keep the immune system strong while also supporting red and white blood cell production.

- Juice of 1 lime
- 1 banana
- 1 mango
- 1/2 jalapeño
- 2 cups cold water (or 1 1/2 cups water plus 1 cup ice)
- 1 tbsp ground flaxseed
- 1 tbsp hemp protein
- 1 tbsp agave nectar
- 1 tbsp hemp oil or EFA Oil Blend (p. 210)

Makes about 3 1/2 cups, or 2 large servings.

Pomegranate Smoothie *(antioxidant-rich)*

raw

This is a simple, refreshing smoothie.

- 1 banana
- 1 date
- 2 cups cold water (or 1 1/2 cups water plus 1 cup ice)
- 1 cup pomegranate seeds (the amount from 1 pomegranate)
- 1 tbsp ground flaxseed
- 1 tbsp hemp protein
- 1 tbsp hemp oil or EFA Oil Blend (p. 210)
- 1/2 tsp cayenne pepper

Makes about 3 1/2 cups, or 2 large servings.

green smoothies

These smoothies are a bit of a departure from the others since they include leafy green vegetables.

Sweet Green Smoothie *(chlorophyll-rich)*

raw

Romaine lettuce is rich in chlorophyll and surprisingly sweet. Blended with melon, it gives this smoothie an especially fresh taste.

6 leaves romaine lettuce
2 fresh or soaked dried dates
2 cups water
1 cup honeydew melon
1 tbsp ground flaxseed
1 tbsp hemp protein
1/2 tbsp grated fresh ginger

Makes about 3 1/2 cups, or 2 large servings.

Kale Calcium Boost Smoothie *(calcium-rich)*

raw

This smoothie is high in calcium thanks to the kale and the sesame seeds of the tahini.

3 leaves kale
1 apple, cored
1 date
2 cups water
1 tbsp ground flaxseed
1 tbsp hemp protein
1 tbsp tahini

Makes about 3 1/2 cups, or 2 large servings.

energy bars

These bars are the healthiest and among the easiest and least time-consuming to prepare. No cooking is required—only a food processor. As you can see from the recipes, these bars are in sharp contrast to commercial energy bars. They are high net-gain bars that don't simply stimulate; they provide nourishment that delivers sustainable energy. I have made these bars for myself since the mid-1990s. In fact, the recipes that follow are what have evolved into the Vega Whole Food Energy Bar that is available in most health food stores and some supermarkets.

Since the moisture content in berries and dates varies slightly, if the mixture is too moist to form into a solid bar, add more of a dry ingredient. If too dry, either add more wet ingredients such as berries or a small amount of water to even it out.

I eat a bar or two a day, so I make a big batch at one time, usually about once a month. I individually wrap each bar and store them in the freezer, easy to grab as I head out the door. Also, these bars will not freeze solid, so you can eat them straight from the freezer—no thawing required. This is an added bonus when taking them along for winter sports, like skiing: These bars stay supple and chewy, whereas many commercial bars freeze solid. On a hot day, a cold bar is as refreshing as ice cream.

You will notice that some of the recipes call for roasted carob powder. As I explain on page 206, the flavor of raw carob is quite mild. If you want the recipe to be 100 percent raw, use cacao nibs (also called raw chocolate) if you can find them. (Be aware that they contain a bit of caffeine.)

Energy Bar Procedure Follow this procedure for all the energy bar recipes, unless otherwise specified:

In a food processor, process all ingredients until desired texture is reached. If you prefer a uniformly smooth bar, process longer. If you would rather a bar with more crunch and texture, blend for less time. Generally, if I'm making them specifically to be eaten during physical activity, such as long training rides, I'll blend the mixture until it is smooth, as this will reduce the amount of chewing required. However, for variety, I'll also be sure to make a few batches at the same time that are crunchier, to eat as a regular snack.

Remove mixture from processor and put on a clean surface. There are two ways to shape the bars: You could roll the mixture into several balls, or shape it into bars.

To shape into balls, use a tablespoon or your hands to scoop the mixture (however much you like to make one ball); roll between the palms of your hands.

To shape as bars, flatten the mixture on the clean surface with your hands. Place plastic wrap over top; with a rolling pin, roll mixture to desired bar thickness. Cut mixture into bars. Alternatively, form mixture into a brick; cut as though slicing bread.

As the bars dry, they become easier to handle.

Chocolate Blueberry Energy Bars

raw option

High in antioxidants and flavonoids, these bars help reduce free radical damage in the body and improve cellular recovery.

1 cup fresh or soaked dried dates
1/4 cup almonds
1/4 cup blueberries
1/4 cup roasted carob powder (or cacao to make 100% raw)
1/4 cup ground flaxseed
1/4 cup hemp protein
1/4 cup unhulled sesame seeds
1 tsp fresh lemon juice
1/2 tsp lemon zest
Sea salt to taste
1/2 cup sprouted or cooked buckwheat (optional)
1/2 cup frozen blueberries

In a food processor, process all ingredients except the buckwheat and blueberries. Knead buckwheat and berries into mixture by hand.

Makes approximately 12 1-3/4 ounce bars.

Ginger Pear Energy Bars

raw

A refreshing, crisp-tasting bar with lots of nutrients and ginger to help fight inflammation and improve digestion.

1 small pear, cored
3/4 cup fresh or soaked dried dates
1/2 cup sunflower seeds

cont.

1/4 cup ground flaxseed
1/4 cup hemp flour
1/4 cup walnuts
2 tbsp grated fresh ginger
Sea salt to taste
2 tbsp sesame seeds

In a food processor, process all ingredients together except the sesame seeds. Cover mixture in sesame seeds before shaping into balls or bars.

Makes approximately 12 1-3/4 ounce bars.

raw

Apple Cinnamon Energy Bars

These bars have a more traditional flavor than the others, yet the same health benefits as a nutrient-dense raw bar.

1 small apple, cored
1 cup fresh or soaked dried dates
1/2 cup soaked or cooked quinoa
1/4 cup almonds
1/4 cup ground flaxseed
1/4 cup hemp flour
2 tsp cinnamon
1/2 tsp nutmeg
Sea salt to taste

Makes approximately 12 1-3/4 ounce bars.

raw option

Spicy Chocolate Energy Bars

These bars offer the taste of chocolate—with a bit of a bite. The macadamia nuts help replace lost electrolytes while the jalapeño pepper creates a feeling of warmth in the body.

1 small banana
1/2 jalapeño
3/4 cup fresh or soaked dried dates
1/2 cup sunflower seeds

cont.

1/4 cup roasted carob powder (or cacao to make 100% raw)
1/4 cup ground flaxseed
1/4 cup macadamia nuts
Sea salt to taste
2 tbsp hemp seeds

In a food processor, process all ingredients together except the hemp seeds. Cover mixture in hemp seeds before shaping into balls or bars.

Makes approximately 12 1-3/4 ounce bars.

Banana Bread Energy Bars

Cinnamon and nutmeg combined with banana give this bar the taste of traditional banana bread, in a healthy, convenient form.

1 small banana
3/4 cup fresh or soaked dried dates
1/2 cup Popped Amaranth (p. 209)
1/2 cup walnuts
1/4 cup ground sesame seeds
2 tsp cinnamon
1/2 tsp nutmeg
Sea salt to taste

Makes approximately 12 1-3/4 ounce bars.

Pomegranate Amaranth Energy Bars

With a refreshing citrus flavor, these energy bars are nut-free and high in antioxidants. They are also exceptionally easy to digest.

3/4 cup fresh or soaked dried dates
1/2 cup pomegranate seeds (the amount from 1/2 pomegranate)
1/2 cup ground flaxseed
1/4 cup hemp seeds
1/4 cup sunflower seeds
1/2 tsp lemon zest
Sea salt to taste
1/4 cup Popped Amaranth (p. 209)

In a food processor, process all ingredients together except amaranth. Remove the mixture from the food processor; work amaranth into it by hand.

Makes approximately 12 1-3/4 ounce bars.

Mango Coconut Energy Bars

raw

With a tropical flavor, high electrolyte content, and energy-producing coconut, these bars are ideal for long physically demanding days.

- 3/4 cup fresh or soaked dried dates
- 1/2 cup chopped mango
- 1/2 cup ground flaxseed
- 1/2 cup soaked or cooked quinoa
- 1/4 cup macadamia nuts
- 1 tsp cinnamon
- 1 tsp lemon zest
- Sea salt to taste
- 1/4 cup shredded coconut

In a food processor, process all ingredients together except coconut. Remove the mixture from the food processor; work coconut into it by hand.

Makes approximately 12 1-3/4 ounce bars.

Citrus Papaya Yerba Maté Energy Bars

For times when you need extra energy, these yerba maté bars will provide it instantly, and their balanced nutrition will keep you going. Since papaya aids in digestion, these are especially good before exercise.

- Zest of 1/2 lemon
- Zest of 1/4 lime
- 2 strips dulse (about 1/4 cup, tightly packed)
- 3/4 cup fresh or soaked dried dates
- 1/2 cup chopped papaya

cont.

1/2 cup Popped Amaranth (p. 209)
1/2 cup ground flaxseed
1/4 cup sunflower seeds
1 tbsp buckwheat flour
2 tsp ground yerba maté
2 tsp agave nectar

Makes approximately 12 1-3/4 ounce bars.

burgers

Thrive Diet burgers are among the fastest and easiest burgers to make, especially when served raw, as these are. They can be made, from start to finish, in about 10 minutes. Although these burgers are delicious and full of nutrition whether raw or cooked, they retain their enzyme content when raw. I opt for the raw version 8 out of 10 times.

I've kept the flavor of these burgers mild so that they readily go with condiments. Topping them with Black Bean Lime Salsa (p. 264) or Mango Chutney (p. 263), or even drizzling them with one of the Thrive Diet salad dressings (recipes begin on page 251) is a good way to dress them up. Also, if you prefer even more flavor, you can substitute the vinegar and the oil component of each recipe with one of the salad dressings. This will instantly infuse the burgers with more flavor. These are hearty, nutrient-dense patties, so one with a mixed-green salad is usually enough for a meal. They can also be served on a whole-wheat bun.

Burger Procedure Follow this procedure for all the burger recipes:

Put all ingredients into a food processor. Process until well blended. Process less if you prefer a coarser texture. Form into 2 patties.

Serve raw or, if you prefer to cook them, lightly cover with coconut oil and bake at 300°F for 35 minutes. Alternatively, lightly fry over medium heat until golden brown, flipping once.

Almond Flaxseed Burger

raw option

- 2 cloves garlic
- 1 cup almonds
- 1/2 cup ground flaxseed
- 2 tbsp balsamic vinegar
- 2 tbsp coconut oil, hemp oil, or EFA Oil Blend (p. 210)
- Sea salt to taste

Makes 2 medium patties.

Walnut Hemp Burger

raw option

- 1 cup walnuts
- 1/2 cup hemp seeds
- 2 tbsp apple cider vinegar
- 2 tbsp coconut oil, hemp oil, or EFA Oil Blend (p. 210)
- 1/2 tsp basil
- 1/2 tsp oregano
- Sea salt to taste

Makes 2 medium patties.

Pecan Sunflower Burger

raw option

- 1 cup pecans
- 1/2 cup ground sunflower seeds
- 2 tbsp apple cider vinegar
- 2 tbsp coconut oil, hemp oil, or EFA Oil Blend (p. 210)
- 1/2 tsp chili flakes
- 1/4 tsp cayenne pepper
- Sea salt to taste

Makes 2 medium patties.

pizzas

I hesitate to even call these pizzas. They bear little resemblance to traditional pizza, other than the way they are served.

Thrive Diet pizza crusts are easy to make and take only a few minutes. Since they are thin crusts, no yeast is needed and therefore they don't need time to rise. Also, since the crusts is wheat-free and gluten-free, no kneading is required. As a result, they are fairly crispy; eating them with a fork and knife is the way to go. The recipes below are packed with nutrition and offer a wide variety of flavor and texture. Some are crispy while others more closely resemble traditional pizza crust. The diversity keeps mealtime interesting.

Each recipe makes enough to cover one standard-size (11-by-15-inch) baking tray.

Not only are these crusts wheat-free, gluten-free, and yeast-free, they are even grain-free. Their base is made with a combination of seeds, legumes, and vegetables, which yields high-density nutrition.

As with the salad dressings and dips, I list hemp oil as the oil of choice in pizza crusts. Hemp is an excellent oil to use; however, as with other recipes, an oil blend is ideal. While hemp oil alone will produce a positive result, the nutritional value is improved by using the EFA Oil Blend (p. 210). Since the pizzas are not cooked above 300°F degrees, oils rich in essential fatty acids will remain in a healthy state.

The toppings that I have paired with each crust are among my favorites. However, they can be altered to suit your own taste. Feel free to swap toppings between recipes and even make creations of your own using this simple pizza-making technique. Vegetables are the base of the Thrive Diet, and so again feel free to use any combination and variety for your creations. If you prefer more vegetables than the recipes call for, simply add more.

As the pizza sauce, I use either the Spicy Sun-Dried Tomato Marinara Sauce (p. 266), or the Sweet Pepper Hemp Pesto (p. 267). These sauces go well with any of the crusts. To add variety, use any of the salad dressings as a pizza sauce. Just blend in ground sunflower seeds, tahini, or even black beans to thicken them. By blending sprouted or cooked black beans or other legumes into the dressings, they take on the texture of a spread and make an intriguing, nutritious pizza sauce. The thickness of the salad dressing will determine the amount of legumes you need to blend in. For most, blend three parts dressing to one part legumes. For a lighter, more neutral taste, try using black-eyed peas instead of black beans—they more readily take on the flavor of the dressing.

To add even more flavor and nutrition to these pizzas, top with Creamy Nutritional Yeast Sauce (p. 262) once out of the oven.

Pizza Procedure Follow this procedure for all the pizza recipes:

Preheat oven to 300°F.

In a food processor, process all crust ingredients until mixture starts to ball up. Lightly oil the baking tray with coconut oil. Spread mixture on tray to about 1/4 inch thick (it can be thicker or thinner if you prefer).

Spread Spicy Sun-Dried Tomato Marinara Sauce (p. 266) or Sweet Pepper Hemp Pesto (p. 267) on crust; add topping.

Bake for 45 minutes. (This will vary slightly depending on the moisture content of the vegetables and the desired crispness of the pizza.)

Spicy Black-Eyed Pea Quinoa Pizza

The crust of this pizza has a smooth, nutty flavor, and a bit of a bite because of the peppers. Nutritionally balanced, it is also filling—it will "stick to you."

Crust

2 cloves garlic

1 cup cooked or sprouted black-eyed peas

1 cup cooked or sprouted quinoa

cont.

1/2 cup chickpea flour
1/4 cup coconut oil, hemp oil, or EFA Oil Blend (p. 210)
1 tsp chili flakes
1/2 tsp black pepper
1/2 tsp cayenne pepper
Sea salt to taste

Topping

1 red bell pepper, sliced
1/2 onion, diced
1/2 medium sweet potato, finely sliced or grated
1 cup cauliflower florets
1/2 cup grated beet
1 tsp chili flakes

Chickpea Curry Pizza

With its mild curry flavor, this pizza crust is nicely complemented by Sweet Pepper Hemp Pesto (p. 267) and topped with sweet potato slices.

Crust

2 cups ground sunflower seeds
1 cup cooked or sprouted chickpeas
1/4 cup coconut oil, hemp oil, or EFA Oil Blend (p. 210)
1 tsp cumin
1 tsp Curry Powder (p. 210)
1/2 tsp turmeric
Sea salt to taste

Topping

1/2 medium sweet potato, finely sliced or grated
1/2 onion, diced
1 cup broccoli florets
1 cup cauliflower florets
1 cup sunflower seed sprouts

Adzuki Bean Quinoa Sesame Pizza

Another heavier crust, this one keeps you full a long time. With its rich assortment of amino acids, it is especially good to eat at the end of a physically demanding day.

Crust

1 cup cooked or sprouted adzuki beans
1 cup cooked or sprouted quinoa
1/2 cup ground sesame seeds
1/4 cup coconut oil, hemp oil, or EFA Oil Blend (p. 210)
2 tbsp dulse flakes

Topping

1 cucumber, sliced
1/2 onion, diced
4 strips dulse (about 1/2 cup tightly packed)
1 cup bean sprouts
1/2 cup chopped fresh basil
1/2 cup chopped green onions

Sunflower Seed Beet Pizza

The crust of this pizza is lighter tasting, with a distinct beet flavor. Beets are alkaline-forming, so this is a good one to make when your stress level is high.

Crust

2 cups ground sunflower seeds
1 cup grated beet
1/4 cup coconut oil, hemp oil, or EFA Oil Blend (p. 210)
1/2 tsp parsley
Sea salt to taste

Topping

1 tomato, sliced
1/2 Spanish onion, diced
1 cup chopped celery
1/2 cup chopped fresh basil
1/2 cup grated carrot
1/2 cup chopped green onions

Sweet Potato Sesame Pizza

This pizza's crust is rich in calcium and phosphorus. It is especially good with Green Tea Miso Gravy (p. 264) used as the sauce.

Crust

1 cup ground sesame seeds
1 cup grated sweet potato
1/2 cup chickpea flour
1/4 cup coconut oil, hemp oil, or EFA Oil Blend (p. 210)
1 tbsp garlic
1 tsp dried basil
Sea salt to taste

Topping

1 tomato, sliced
1/2 onion, diced
1 cup chopped red bell peppers
1/2 cup grated beet
1/2 cup chopped green onions
1 tsp oregano (or 1 tbsp fresh)
1 tsp thyme (or 1 tbsp fresh)

Chili Kidney Bean Pizza

A particularly filling pizza, this one will keep you going strong for hours.

Crust

1 1/2 cups cooked brown rice
1 1/2 cups kidney beans
1/4 cup coconut oil, hemp oil, or EFA Oil Blend (p. 210)
1 tbsp chili powder
1 tsp chili flakes
Sea salt to taste

Topping

1 tomato, sliced
1/2 onion, diced
1 cup chopped bell peppers (any color)

cont.

1/2 cup grated carrot
1/2 cup chopped green onions
1 tsp oregano (or 1 tbsp fresh)
1 tsp thyme (or 1 tbsp fresh)

Curry Lentil Rice Pizza

This recipe features the familiar combination of curry, lentils, and rice in a form it's not usually found—pizza crust.

Crust

1 1/2 cups cooked brown rice
1 1/2 cups ground lentils
1/4 cup coconut oil, hemp oil, or EFA Oil Blend (p. 210)
2 tsp Curry Powder (p. 210)
1 tsp basil
Sea salt to taste

Topping

1 tomato, sliced
1/2 Spanish onion, diced
1 cup chopped celery
1 cup chopped red bell peppers
1/2 cup grated carrot
1/2 cup chopped green onions
1 tsp oregano (or 1 tbsp fresh)
1 tsp thyme (or 1 tbsp fresh)

Popped Amaranth Rooibos Pizza

This pizza is one of the lighter Thrive Diet pizzas.

Crust

2 cups Popped Amaranth (p. 209)
1 cup cooked or sprouted red lentils
1/4 cup coconut oil, hemp oil, or EFA Oil Blend (p. 210)
1 tbsp ground rooibos
Sea salt to taste

cont.

Topping

1 tomato, sliced
1 cup chopped yellow bell pepper
1 cup chopped snow peas
1/2 cup grated beet
1/2 cup chopped cilantro
1/2 cup chopped green onions
1 tsp oregano (or 1 tbsp fresh)
1 tsp thyme (or 1 tbsp fresh)

Wild Rice Split Pea Pizza

I eat this pizza mostly in the autumn; it just seems to fit with the season.

Crust

1 1/2 cups cooked split yellow peas
1 1/2 cups cooked or sprouted wild rice
1/4 cup coconut oil, hemp oil, or EFA Oil Blend (p. 210)
2 tsp basil
1 tsp thyme
Sea salt to taste

Topping

1/2 red onion, diced
1 cup chopped broccoli florets
1/2 cup chopped green onions
1/2 cup grated parsnip
1 tsp basil (or 1 tbsp fresh)
1 tsp oregano (or 1 tbsp fresh)
1 tsp thyme (or 1 tbsp fresh)

vegetables

Packed with vitamins and minerals, these delicious vegetable dishes can be eaten as a meal in themselves or as a side dish with soup and salad.

Ginger Lime Squash

raw option

To make this a raw dish, substitute an uncooked, finely grated sweet potato or even a zucchini for the squash.

- 2 cups peeled and cubed (bite-size) squash
- 2 green onions
- 1 clove garlic
- 1/2 cup chopped or torn cilantro
- 2 tbsp hemp oil
- 1 tbsp fresh lime juice
- 1/2 to 1 tbsp finely chopped ginger
- 1/4 tsp chili flakes

Steam or boil the cubed squash. Meanwhile, finely chop the green onions and the garlic (or use a garlic press).

Let the squash cool. In a bowl, combine all ingredients. For the best flavor, allow to refrigerate for a few hours or overnight.

Makes 2 servings.

Dinosaur Kale Quinoa Wrap

raw option

As a meal or appetizer, this nutrient-dense wrap is surprisingly filling. For the dressing, choose one of the Thrive Diet dressings; recipes begin on page 251. The Balsamic Vinaigrette (p. 256) goes particularly well.

- 1 avocado
- 2 Roma tomatoes
- 1 cucumber
- 1 large carrot
- 2 strips dulse (about 1/4 cup, tightly packed)
- 1 cup soaked or cooked quinoa
- 1 leaf dinosaur kale
- 3 tbsp salad dressing

Peel and cube avocado, slice tomatoes and cucumber, and grate carrot. Place, along with the dulse and quinoa, on a leaf of kale.

Drizzle salad dressing over top. Roll up, tucking ends in so the wrap is secure. Cut into pieces if desired.

Variation: To serve as a complete meal, add 1/2 cup black-eyed peas and 1/2 tsp cayenne pepper to the mixture to spice it up.

Dinosaur kale also serves as a good wrap for guacamole combined with either quinoa, popped amaranth, or brown rice.

Makes 1 meal-size serving or 3 appetizer-size servings.

Lemon Ginger Plantain with Dulse

The sugar of the plantain caramelizes and blends with the citrus from the lemon to make for an intriguing, refreshing treat. The riper the plantain, the sweeter it will be. The mineral salt in the dulse really brings out the flavor. Turning crispy when fried, the dulse strips add crunch. Add ginger for a sharper taste. This dish is a nice accompaniment to any salad.

- 1 plantain
- 4 strips dulse (about 3/4 cup, tightly packed)
- 1 tbsp coconut oil
- 1 tbsp fresh lemon juice
- 1/2 tbsp finely chopped or grated fresh ginger (optional)

Peel and thinly slice plantain on an angle. Heat coconut oil in frying pan over medium heat. Lightly stir-fry plantain slices until slightly brown. Stir in lemon juice and dulse strips (and ginger if using). Stir-fry until juice has evaporated and dulse is crispy.

Makes 1 serving.

Crunchy Cinnamon Plantain Strips

As strips or broken into chips, these are great crunchy snacks, full of complementary flavor. They can be eaten on their own or with a pâté in place of crackers. The Sunflower Seed Pâté (p. 266) is a perfect match.

- 1 large plantain
- 1/2 tbsp coconut oil
- 1 tsp fresh lemon juice

cont.

1/2 tsp cinnamon

1/4 tsp sea salt

Preheat oven to 300°F.

Peel and thinly slice plantain from end to end; the strips should be long. Place on a baking tray lightly oiled with coconut oil.

If coconut oil is hard, heat until liquid. Combine lemon juice with coconut oil.

Rub a bit of oil and juice mixture on top of each plantain strip. Rub on cinnamon and sea salt.

Bake for 25 minutes.

Makes 1 serving.

Zucchini Pasta

raw option

Instead of eating starchy, gluten-based pasta, try a raw zucchini one. This can be eaten later in the evening without any concern of packing on the pounds. Plus, it is very easily digested so will not have your digestive system working overtime while you sleep. This "pasta" goes especially well with Spicy Sun-Dried Tomato Marinara Sauce (p. 266).

Other vegetables, including carrots and beets, can be substituted for the zucchini, but they have a more pronounced flavor and may overpower the sauce.

1 zucchini

Use a vegetable peeler to peel the zucchini into strips.

For added flavor and variety, lightly stir-fry with a few flavorful ingredients.

3/4 tbsp coconut oil

1 small clove garlic, finely chopped

1 cup soaked arame

1 tbsp sesame seeds

Heat coconut oil in a frying pan or wok over medium heat. Add garlic and lightly brown. Add the arame and sesame seeds. Stir-fry for about

3 minutes or until desired texture is reached. The longer it is stir-fried, the crispier the strips will become. Remove from heat and top with sauce.

Makes 1 serving.

Garlic Oregano Yam Oven Fries

An good addition to a salad, these fries are almost a meal in themselves. This recipe is one of the healthiest ways to prepare yams. Or dip them in Ketchup (p. 261).

2 medium yams
2 cloves garlic
2 tbsp coarsely chopped pumpkin seeds
1 tbsp oregano
1 1/2 tbsp coconut oil
1/2 tbsp basil
Sea salt to taste

Preheat oven to 300°F.

Cut yams into wedges or chunks. In bowl, combine the garlic, pumpkin seeds, oregano, coconut oil, basil, and sea salt. Add the yams, stirring with your hands to making sure all the pieces are covered with the mixture. Spread yams on a baking tray lightly oiled with coconut oil; bake for about 35 minutes. If you prefer them crispier, leave in oven for an extra 5 to 10 minutes.

Makes 2 servings.

soups

These soups are quick and easy to prepare: No cooking required. The friction created by the blender will heat the soup to slightly above room temperature. While you may choose to heat these soups further on the stove, be sure to not exceed about 110°F, since that's the point at which heat will begin to destroy the enzymes. These soups are especially refreshing served chilled as part of a light summer meal. They all go well with any of the crackers (recipes begin on page 257).

Sesame Miso Soup

raw option

This alkalizing soup, rich in calcium and trace minerals, provides natural-source electrolytes to help restore balance in the body after exercise.

- 2 cups water
- 3 strips dulse (about 1/3 cup, tightly packed)
- 1 medium scallion, finely chopped
- 2 tbsp ground unhulled sesame seeds
- 2 tbsp brown rice miso paste

In a pot, heat water over medium heat; add dulse, scallion, sesame seeds, and miso paste.

Variations: For a more intense flavor, lightly stir-fry the scallion and the ground sesame seeds in 1 tbsp coconut oil. Black sesame seeds are also a nice variation from the usual white variety. For added nutrition, add 1 tbsp hemp protein.

Makes 2 small servings.

Creamy Ginger Carrot Soup

raw

This is an especially easy soup to digest. Because of the ginger, it has a warming effect whether served warm or cold.

- 3 large carrots
- 1 avocado, pit and skin removed
- 2 cups water
- 1 1/2 tsp grated ginger
- Sea salt to taste
- 1/4 cup coarsely chopped or torn cilantro

Grate carrots. In a food processor, process avocado and water. Once smooth, add carrots, ginger, and sea salt. Process to desired consistency. Stir in cilantro and serve.

Makes 2 servings.

Creamy Pepper Soup

raw

A refreshing, nutrient-packed soup, this one is best served cold on a warm day.

1 avocado, pit and skin removed
1 red or yellow bell pepper
2 cups water or Hemp Milk (p. 268)
1/4 cup chopped cilantro
1/2 tsp dulse flakes
Pinch of oregano

In a food processor, process all ingredients together.

Makes 2 servings.

Green Soup

raw

This is an excellent summertime soup, packed with naturally occurring electrolytes and enzymes.

1/2 avocado, pit and skin removed
3 cups water
2 cups spinach, tightly packed
1/2 cup chopped parsley
2 tbsp hemp protein
2 tbsp pumpkin seeds
1 tbsp hemp oil
1/2 tbsp grated fresh ginger
1 tsp fresh lemon juice
1/4 tsp ground stevia leaf

In a food processor, process all ingredients together.

Makes 2 large servings.

salads

Since the Thrive Diet is built on greens and other vegetables, a big salad is part of each day's meal plan, often as a main course. These recipes are not for your run-of-the-mill salad—they are for satisfying, nutrient-packed meals.

Below I've listed the primary ingredients that I use in about 90 percent of my salads. There is no wrong way to combine these ingredients; they are all nutritional powerhouses. With each salad recipe, I suggest the dressing that I have found best complements it, in taste and nutritionally—the ingredients work together synergistically, making for an even greater result.

Most supermarkets carry prewashed mixed greens. I use these as the base for most of my salads since they offer variety. However, you may choose to create your own combination. In the recipe, the greens are measured in cups; this is based on tightly packed cups. Of course, it is a guide only and you don't need to follow it strictly. The proportions of each ingredient in the salads are flexible. If you want more of a particular ingredient, add more.

Most health food stores and supermarkets sell sprouts in the produce department. They are a healthy addition to any salad. One caution: Since bacteria can develop in fresh sprouts, people with a compromised immune system may want to avoid store-bought sprouts.

Main Thrive Diet Salad Ingredients:

Mixed greens:
- Beet greens
- Butter lettuce
- Collards
- Dandelion greens
- Dinosaur kale
- Kale
- Mustard greens
- Red leaf lettuce
- Romaine lettuce
- Spinach
- Swiss chard

Almonds
Amaranth (popped) (p. 209)
Avocado
Beet
Bell peppers
Black beans
Carrots
Cucumbers

Dulse strips
Hemp seeds
Legumes (sprouted) (p. 203)
Nori
Nutritional yeast
Pumpkin seeds
Quinoa
Snow peas
Sugar snap peas
Sunflower seed sprouts

Salad Procedure Follow this procedure for all the salad recipes, unless otherwise specified:

Wash greens (unless already prewashed). In a bowl, combine all ingredients. Top with dressing.

To make any of these salads 100% raw, leave out the nutritional yeast, popped amaranth, or baked ingredient (e.g., crackers) if called for.

Avocado Cayenne Salad

raw

Suggested dressing: Balsamic Vinaigrette (p. 256)

The satiating quality of avocado combined with B vitamin–rich nori and nutritional yeast makes this salad a good one for sustaining an even energy level. The cayenne helps improve circulation, warming the body and making this a good wintertime salad.

1/2 avocado, sliced
1 sheet nori, chopped
4 cups mixed greens
1 tbsp nutritional yeast
1/2 tsp cayenne pepper

Crunchy Cinnamon Plantain and Macadamia Nut Salad

raw option

Suggested dressing: Mango Lime Dressing (p. 254)

High in trace minerals, the plantain and the dulse in this salad help replenish the body's electrolytes after higher-than-usual levels of sweat loss—great for after a long workout or Bikram's yoga class, or even just on a warm summer evening. Because of their healthy fats, protein, and fiber, the macadamia nuts give this salad staying power and a good dose of potassium, a prime electrolyte lost in sweat.

4 cups mixed greens
1 cup sunflower seed sprouts
1/2 cup chopped sugar snap peas
1/2 cup bite-size pieces of Crunchy Cinnamon Plantain Strips (p. 242)
1/4 cup chopped dulse
2 tbsp chopped macadamia nuts

Cucumber Dill Salad

Suggested dressing: Cucumber Dill Dressing (p. 256)

The Curry Lentil Crackers in this salad provide sustenance, while the sunflower seeds supply a good dose of selenium and vitamin E, both powerful antioxidants. The coolness of the dill nicely complements the curry's warming effect.

1/2 cucumber, grated
4 cups mixed greens
1/2 cup grated carrot
1/2 cup bite-size pieces of Curry Lentil Crackers (p. 259)
1/4 cup chopped dulse
2 tbsp sunflower seeds

Popped Amaranth Hemp Seed Salad

raw option

Suggested dressing: Cayenne Dill Tahini Dressing (p. 253)

Hemp seeds combined with amaranth give this salad an exceptional protein profile.

1 sheet nori, chopped
4 cups mixed greens
1/2 cup Popped Amaranth (p. 209)
1/2 cup chopped snow peas
2 tbsp hemp seeds

Lemon Crisp Beet Salad

raw option

Suggested dressing: Orange Pumpkin Seed Dressing (p. 255)

Iron-rich kale and pumpkin seeds combine with the vitamin C in the lemon crisps (and the Orange Pumpkin Seed Dressing, if used) in this salad to keep the blood healthy by helping build red blood cells.

1 leaf dinosaur kale
2 dulse strips (about 1/4 cup, tightly packed)
3 cups mixed greens
1/2 cup grated beet
1/2 cup bite-size pieces of Lemon Sesame Crisps (p. 260)
2 tbsp pumpkin seeds

Creamy Carrot Salad

raw option

Suggested dressing: Macadamia Dill Dressing (p. 255)

Calcium-rich dinosaur kale and the sesame seeds in the Nutritional Yeast and Sesame Seed Topping make this salad especially calcium rich and therefore alkaline-forming. If bone health is a concern, this salad is a practical dietary solution. Also plentiful in B vitamins from the nutritional yeast and sprouts, this salad helps the body burn carbohydrate more efficiently.

1 leaf dinosaur kale
1/2 cup grated carrot
3 cups mixed greens
1 cup sunflower seed sprouts
3 tbsp Nutritional Yeast and Sesame Seed Topping (p. 211)

Zucchini Chip Almond Salad

raw option

Suggested dressing: Pomegranate Poppy Seed Dressing (p. 257)

Because of the soaked almonds and red pepper, this salad is particularly high in antioxidants. The Zucchini Chips provide a good source of electrolytes, making this a good salad to replenish and repair the body.

1/2 cucumber, grated
4 cups mixed greens
1/2 cup sliced red peppers
1/2 cup bite-size pieces of Zucchini Chips (p. 260)
2 tbsp soaked and chopped almonds

Cucumber Pesto Salad

raw option

Suggested dressing: Tomato Basil Dressing (p. 256)

In part because of the garlic, this salad is a good immune booster. If you eat this salad at the first sign of a cold, you may find that the cold never materializes. The high vitamin K content in the pine nuts helps prevent blood clots.

1/2 clove garlic, chopped
1/2 cucumber, grated
4 cups mixed greens
3 tbsp Nutritional Yeast and Sesame Seed Topping (p. 211)
2 tbsp pine nuts

Arame Seaweed Salad

Suggested dressing: Any of the dressing recipes in this book can be used instead of the hemp oil and lemon juice listed below.

Arame seaweed is a good introduction to sea vegetables for those who are unaccustomed to them. It has a mild flavor that does not have as strong a taste of the sea as some other sea vegetables do. As with most sea vegetables, arame is a rich source of iodine and calcium, and it is alkaline-forming.

2 cups arame seaweed
2 tbsp unhulled sesame seeds (or hemp seeds)
1 tbsp hemp oil
2 tsp fresh lemon juice

Soak arame in water for about 20 minutes; 15 minutes is enough if you prefer a slightly crunchy texture. Mix all ingredients together.

Variation: Add 2 tsp agave nectar and 1/8 tsp cayenne pepper for a sweet, hot flavor.

salad dressings

Green salads are among the healthiest of foods. Why, then, don't most salad dressings mirror their health-promoting qualities? Not one commercial salad dressing fit Thrive Diet parameters. Many are based on low-quality processed oil, and most contain refined sugar.

The price of commercial salad dressings varies greatly depending on the type of oil used.

The cheaper varieties generally use a base of cottonseed, palm, or safflower oil. Soybean, canola, and olive oil–based dressings are one level better, yet still far from ideal. Extra-virgin olive oil is generally the best oil source found in commercial salad dressing.

The processing of oil—the way in which the oil is extracted from the seed, olive, or whatever the primary source may be—can be the difference between good and bad. Some extraction methods for cheaper oils involve high heat, which can actually cause the oil to convert to trans fat. Other extraction methods use chemical solvents to separate the oil, usually done with low-grade oils. When selecting oils, be sure to choose ones that are labeled "cold pressed" or "raw." This will ensure that the proper measures have been taken when extracting the oils to maintain the integrity of the oil. Don't assume that most salad dressings are raw—most are heat processed.

Quality is often compromised when low-quality oils are processed. To increase shelf life and prevent the oil from becoming rancid once bottled, heavy solvents are often used. Since taste and smell are altered by the use of these chemicals, the oil is then heated to high temperature, to eliminate any unpleasant odor and taste left by the processing procedure. Oils that have been through that process are particularly unhealthy and should adamantly be avoided. Unfortunately, many commercial dressings, dips, and spreads include ingredients that have been subjected to this treatment.

Since I eat at least one big salad a day and base the Thrive Diet on greens, I found I needed several good salad dressings, for variety. My recipes are designed for their health-promoting ingredients as much as they are for taste. Because of their nutrient-rich properties, using these dressings with other foods is a good way to enrich their value also. Since oil is obtained from a seed, its nutrition value often very closely parallels the nutrition of the seed itself or plant that it would grow into. However, the oil is in a highly concentrated form and therefore offers a wealth of intense nourishment.

Blending ground sunflower seeds, black beans, or black-eyed peas into the dressings will thicken them so they also can be used as dips, spreads, and sauces. Try them as a pizza crust sauce, a burger topping, a dip for Garlic Oregano Yam Oven Fries (p. 244) or raw vegetables, and even as a sauce on Zucchini Pasta (p. 243).

Feel free to experiment with dressings of your own, too. As long as the base consists of a high-quality oil such as hemp oil or, better yet, the EFA Oil Blend (p. 210), along with a high-quality vinegar such as balsamic or apple cider, you can't go wrong. Lemon juice is another high-quality base ingredient.

Salad Dressing Procedure Follow this procedure for all the salad dressing recipes, unless otherwise specified:

In a blender, blend all ingredients together. The flavors will take up to a day to combine completely. I make a bottle of three or four flavors and store in the refrigerator to have them on hand; they stay fresh for up to a month.

Cayenne Dill Tahini Dressing

raw

This is a full-flavored dressing with a bit of bite. The tahini offers a good amount of calcium, and the cayenne pepper helps get the blood flowing.

- 1/2 clove garlic
- 1/2 cup balsamic vinegar
- 1/2 cup hemp oil or EFA Oil Blend (p. 210)
- 1/4 cup water
- 2 tbsp tahini
- 1/2 tbsp dill
- 1/2 tsp cayenne pepper
- 1/4 tsp agave nectar
- Sea salt to taste

Makes about 1 1/2 cups.

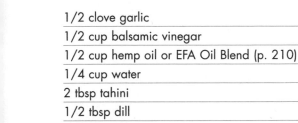

Creamy Ginger Dressing

This is a thick, creamy dressing with a strong flavor. Only a small amount needs to be used on salad to boost its flavor. By doubling the amount of tahini and nutritional yeast, it can also serve as a dip for Garlic Oregano Yam Oven Fries (p. 244), or be drizzled over a burger.

As with all recipes containing nutritional yeast, it is high in B vitamins. With the ginger, it is also helps reduce inflammation and aids in digestion, making it especially good to have with cooked food.

1/2 cup hemp oil or EFA Oil Blend (p. 210)
2 tbsp apple cider vinegar
2 tbsp tahini
2 tbsp water
2 tsp grated fresh ginger
2 tsp nutritional yeast
Sea salt to taste

Makes about 1 1/2 cups.

raw

Mango Lime Dressing

A sweet dressing with a bit of a bite, this one is particularly good on burgers. If you like, papaya can be substituted for the mango.

1 mango
1/4 jalapeño
1/4 cup fresh lime juice
1 tbsp hemp oil or EFA Oil Blend (p. 210)
1 tbsp lime zest
1 tsp agave nectar

Makes about 1 1/2 cups.

raw

Ginger Carrot Dressing

With its light, fresh flavor, this dressing is versatile.

1/2 cup apple cider vinegar
1/4 cup shredded carrot

cont.

1/4 cup hemp oil or EFA Oil Blend (p. 210)
2 tsp grated fresh ginger
1/2 tsp fresh lime juice

Makes about 1 cup.

raw

Orange Pumpkin Seed Dressing

This is a light vinaigrette with a slightly sweet-and-sour taste. The orange juice makes it sweet, while the apple cider vinegar and pumpkin seeds give it a hint of bitterness. This dressing provides an iron boost: The vitamin C in the orange juice helps with absorption of the iron from the pumpkin seeds.

1/2 cup orange juice
1/4 cup hemp oil or EFA Oil Blend (p. 210)
1 tbsp pumpkin seeds
1 tsp orange zest
1 tsp apple cider vinegar
Sea salt to taste

Makes about 1 cup.

raw

Macadamia Dill Dressing

A creamy, sweet dressing, this one is also good as a dip and a burger sauce.

1/2 cup macadamia nuts
1/4 cup plus 1 tbsp apple cider vinegar
4 tsp dried dill (or 2 tbsp fresh)
2 tsp agave nectar
Black pepper and sea salt to taste

Makes about 1 cup.

Caesar Dressing

This rich, satisfying dressing greatly complements simple greens.

1 clove garlic
1/3 stalk green onion

cont.

3/4 cup hemp oil or EFA Oil Blend (p. 210)
1/4 cup macadamia nuts
2 tbsp brown rice miso paste
1 1/2 tbsp apple cider vinegar
1 1/2 tbsp fresh lemon juice
2 tsp nutritional yeast
1/4 tsp cayenne pepper

Makes about 1 1/2 cups.

Tomato Basil Dressing

raw

2 tomatoes
2 tbsp apple cider vinegar
2 tbsp hemp oil or EFA Oil Blend (p. 210)
1 tbsp dried basil (or 3 tbsp fresh)
1 tbsp agave nectar
Black pepper and sea salt to taste

Makes about 1 1/2 cups.

Balsamic Vinaigrette

raw

A classic.

6 cloves garlic
1 cup hemp oil or EFA Oil Blend (p. 210)
1/2 cup balsamic vinegar

Makes about 1 1/2 cups.

Cucumber Dill Dressing

raw

A simple fresh dressing, also good to drizzle over Garlic Oregano Yam Oven Fries (p. 243). You can either process this dressing until it's smooth, or, if you prefer the cucumber to be a bit chunky, process just a few seconds less.

4 cloves garlic
2 cucumbers, peeled

cont.

1/2 cup hemp oil or EFA Oil Blend (p. 210)
4 tsp dried dill (or 4 tbsp fresh)
Black pepper and sea salt to taste

Makes about 2 cups.

Pomegranate Poppy Seed Dressing

raw

A high-antioxidant dressing, particularly refreshing on a warm day.

3 tbsp pomegranate juice
2 tbsp hemp oil or EFA Oil Blend (p. 210)
1 tbsp agave nectar
1 tbsp apple cider vinegar
1 tsp lemon zest
Sea salt to taste
1/2 cup pomegranate seeds (the amount from 1/2 pomegranate)
1 tbsp poppy seeds

In a food processor, process the pomegranate juice, oil, agave nectar, apple cider vinegar, lemon zest, and sea salt until smooth. Add the pomegranate seeds and poppy seeds; pulse a couple of times until the seeds are broken but not completely blended in.

Makes about 2 cups.

crackers

These crackers go well with salsa, guacamole, and dips. They are also a good addition to salads in place of traditional croutons. They add texture and, of course, high-quality nutrition.

Since these crackers keep well, I make a large batch once a month or so, storing them in an open container in the refrigerator.

Cracker Procedure Follow this procedure for all the cracker recipes, unless otherwise specified:

Preheat oven to 300°F.

In a food processor, process all ingredients. Lightly oil a baking tray with coconut oil. Spread mixture on baking tray as thinly as possible. (Or, if you prefer slightly thicker crackers, don't spread as thin and bake for about 10 minutes longer.) Each recipe makes enough dough to fill approximately one standard-size (11-by-15-inch) baking tray. Score mixture with a knife to mark desired cracker size before baking.

Bake for 30 minutes. Remove from oven; let cool.

Lemon Rooibos Crackers

These high-antioxidant crackers have a slightly sweet-and-sour flavor. They go well with Sweet Pepper Hemp Pesto (p. 267).

1/4 cup almonds
1/4 cup pecans
1/4 cup sesame seeds
3 tbsp fresh lemon juice
1 tbsp lemon zest
1 tbsp coconut oil
1 tsp ground rooibos
1/2 tsp agave nectar
Sea salt to taste

Makes 2 servings.

Green Tea Ginger Lime Crackers

These crackers offer just a hint of ginger and a slight citrus zing from the lime. They go particularly well with the Miso Kelp Guacamole (p. 263) and Black Bean Lime Salsa (p. 264).

1/4 cup almonds
1/4 cup Popped Amaranth (p. 209)
1/4 cup sunflower seeds
3 tbsp fresh lime juice
1 1/2 tbsp lime zest
1 tbsp coconut oil
1/2 tbsp grated fresh ginger

cont.

1 tsp finely ground green tea leaves (or 1/2 tsp matcha powder)
1/2 tsp agave nectar
Sea salt to taste

Makes 2 servings.

Curry Lentil Crackers

A meal in themselves, these crackers combined with Pineapple Salsa (p. 265) or Black-Eyed Pea Cayenne Salsa (p. 265) will deliver a large amount of nutrition in a compact form.

1/4 cup chickpea flour
1/4 cup cooked or sprouted lentils
1/4 cup ground sunflower seeds
2 tbsp balsamic vinegar
1 tbsp coconut oil
2 tsp Curry Powder (p. 210)
1 tsp cumin
1/2 tsp agave nectar
Sea salt to taste

Makes 2 servings.

Vegetable Crackers

Particularly good with Sunflower Seed Pâté (p. 266), these vegetable crackers are a flavorful snack.

1 1/2 cups ground flaxseed
1/2 cup chopped celery
1/2 cup chopped tomato
1/2 cup almonds
1/2 cup sunflower seeds
1/4 cup chopped carrot
1 tsp cumin
Sea salt to taste

Makes 2 servings.

Zucchini Chips

These chips go well with salsa, nut butters, and guacamole. Their mild flavor allows others to shine through. Zucchini chips are also a crunchy treat just on their own. They are a good alternative to croutons in a salad.

2 zucchini
1 tbsp coconut oil
Sea salt to taste

Peel zucchini; cut into thin strips. (Alternatively, the zucchini can be sliced into thin "chips.") Place on a baking tray lightly oiled with extra coconut oil. Rub coconut oil and salt on top of each strip.

Bake for 30 minutes.

Variation: For a late-night snack, add herbs to add flavor. Or, for a sweeter taste, use 1/2 tsp ground stevia leaf instead of the herbs.

1 tbsp coconut oil
1/2 tsp thyme
1/4 tsp basil
1/4 tsp oregano

Melt the coconut oil over medium heat. Stir in thyme, basil, and oregano. Coat zucchini chips with oil mixture before baking.

Makes 1 serving.

Lemon Sesame Crisps

I developed these as an everyday snack, but they're also great to eat while exercising. Their crispy texture is a good contrast to the softer foods and gels usually eaten during exercise. I take a pack of these simple, refreshing crisps with me for my longer, less intense workouts. The sesame seeds provide calcium, needed during long bouts of exercise to help maintain smooth muscle contractions. Dulse replenishes the electrolytes lost in sweat.

2/3 cup sesame seeds
1/3 cup agave nectar
1/4 cup lemon zest
2 tbsp dulse flakes

cont.

2 tbsp coconut oil

2 tbsp fresh lemon juice

Preheat oven to 300°F.

In a food processor, mix all ingredients together. Lightly oil baking tray with extra coconut oil. Spread mixture over baking tray to desired thickness. Score mixture with a knife to mark desired crisp size.

Bake for 20 minutes. Remove from oven and let cool and harden before breaking up.

Variation: Substitute hemp seeds for the sesame seeds and a lime for the lemon, for a different flavor.

If you choose to make the crisps to eat during exercise and you want a bit of an extra kick, add 1 tbsp ground yerba maté to the mixture, plus an extra 1/2 tbsp agave nectar.

Makes 2 servings.

sauces, dips, and spreads

These sauces, dips, and spreads complement whatever they accompany, rather than masking the taste, as many commercial products do. They are all highly nutritious: their addition to a meal or snack will fortify it with protein, essential fatty acids, and fiber.

Ketchup

raw

I went for years without eating ketchup, until I started making my own. Commercial ketchups are full of refined sugar. Also, when tomatoes are heated to high temperatures, as the commercial ones are in processing, many of their disease-fighting properties as well as enzymes are reduced. This recipe is raw, so all the health-promoting benefits of the whole foods remain intact.

4 fresh or soaked dried dates

1 cup chopped tomato

1 cup sun-dried tomatoes

cont.

1/4 cup chopped onion
1/4 cup agave nectar
1/4 cup hemp oil or EFA Oil Blend (p. 210)
2 tbsp apple cider vinegar
1 tsp oregano
Sea salt to taste

In a food processor, process all ingredients until smooth. Keep refrigerated for up to 4 weeks.

Makes about 3 cups.

Creamy Nutritional Yeast Sauce

This sauce quite closely resembles melted cheese in both texture and taste. It is great as a topping on burgers, as a dip, or even for mixing with guacamole for an extra-flavorful dip or condiment. It can also be added to pizza.

The nutritional yeast delivers a full spectrum of B vitamins and trace minerals and, combined with the other ingredients, makes for a nutrient-dense sauce.

1 1/2 cups water
1 cup nutritional yeast flakes
1/2 cup sunflower seeds
1 tbsp apple cider vinegar
1 tbsp hemp oil or EFA Oil Blend (p. 210)
1 tsp paprika
1/4 tsp cayenne pepper
1/4 tsp sea salt

Mix all ingredients in a bowl. Heat a frying pan over low heat. Pour mixture into pan; stir continually for 3 to 5 minutes until sauce thickens. The longer the sauce is left on the heat, the thicker it will become. Remove from heat just before mixture has reached the desired thickness, as it will thicken slightly once removed from the heat.

This sauce will keep in the refrigerator for up to 1 week but is best when served fresh.

Makes about 2 cups.

Mango Chutney

This chutney complements many Thrive Diet recipes—try it as a chip dip, especially with Curry Lentil Crackers (p. 259), as a burger topping, or even as an addition to pizza.

7 large fresh or soaked dried dates
1/2 cup water
2 large mangos
1 clove garlic, minced
1/4 cup apple cider vinegar
1 tbsp grated fresh ginger
1 tbsp coconut oil
1/4 tsp cayenne pepper
1/4 tsp sea salt

Mince 3 of the dates. In a food processor, blend the 4 remaining dates with 1/2 cup water. Peel and dice the mangos. Heat a frying pan over low heat and add all ingredients. Simmer for 25 minutes.

Keep refrigerated for up to 1 week.

Makes about 2 1/2 cups.

Miso Kelp Guacamole

raw

This guacamole goes well on burgers, wrapped in dinosaur kale, or with crackers.

2 well-ripened avocados, pit and skin removed
1/2 diced tomato
1 clove garlic, minced
1/4 cup finely chopped kelp
1/4 cup minced onion
1/4 cup tahini
3 tbsp brown rice miso paste
1 1/2 tbsp fresh lemon juice

Mash all ingredients together or process in a food processor.

Keep refrigerated for up to 1 week (it will turn brown but this isn't harmful).

Makes about 2 cups.

Green Tea Miso Gravy

This flavorful gravy delivers probiotics for digestive health.

- 2 tbsp coconut oil
- 1 onion, diced
- 3 tbsp ground sesame seeds
- 1 tsp finely ground green tea leaves (or 1/2 tsp matcha powder)
- 1 cup brewed green tea
- 1 1/2 tbsp brown rice miso paste

Heat coconut oil in frying pan over medium heat. Add onion and ground sesame seeds, and lightly fry. Add the ground tea leaves, brewed green tea, and miso paste; stir well.

Keep refrigerated for up to 1 week.

Makes about 2 cups.

Black Bean Lime Salsa

raw

With its citrus bite, this is one of my favorite salsas. For a summer dinner, I'll have this with Curry Lentil Crackers (p. 259) as my main course. It is refreshing, yet provides balanced sustenance. The salsa also works well on burgers or as a dip for Vegetable Crackers (p. 259).

- Juice of 1/2 lime
- 2 cloves garlic, finely chopped
- 1 tomato, diced
- 1/2 onion, diced
- 1 cup black beans
- 1 cup coarsely chopped or torn cilantro
- 1 tbsp balsamic vinegar
- 1 tbsp hemp oil
- 1/2 tsp cayenne pepper
- 1/4 tsp sea salt

In a bowl, combine all ingredients. Allow to sit for a few hours at room temperature so that the flavors infuse.

Keep refrigerated for up to 1 week.

Makes about 2 cups.

Black-Eyed Pea Cayenne Salsa

raw option

A spicy, nourishing salsa that goes well with Curry Lentil Crackers (p. 259). Or try wrapping in a leaf of dinosaur kale.

- Juice of 1 lemon
- 1 tomato, diced
- 1/2 onion, diced
- 1 cup black-eyed peas
- 1 cup coarsely chopped or torn cilantro
- 1 tbsp balsamic vinegar
- 1 tbsp hemp oil
- 1/2 tsp cayenne pepper
- 1/2 tsp chili flakes
- 1/4 tsp sea salt

In a bowl, combine all ingredients. Allow to sit for a few hours at room temperature so that the flavors infuse.

Keep refrigerated for up to 1 week.

Makes about 2 cups.

Pineapple Salsa

raw

This salsa is a nice alternative to the usual tomato variety.

- 1/2 jalapeño, chopped
- 2 cups cubed pineapple
- 1/2 cup chopped red bell pepper
- 1/4 cup diced Spanish onion
- 1 tbsp chopped cilantro

cont.

1 tbsp fresh lime juice
1 tbsp hemp oil
1 tsp lime zest

In a food processor, process all ingredients until a consistent texture.

Keep refrigerated for up to 1 week.

Makes about 3 cups.

Sunflower Seed Pâté

raw

This mild pâté is a great accompaniment to flavored crackers.

2 cloves garlic
2 cups sunflower seeds
1/2 cup walnuts
1/3 cup hemp oil
1/4 cup orange juice
1 tsp sea salt

In a food processor, process all ingredients together until smooth.

Keep refrigerated for up to 2 weeks.

Makes about 2 cups.

Spicy Sun-Dried Tomato Marinara Sauce

raw

Thanks to the sun-dried tomatoes, this sauce is full of flavor. It is tasty as a sauce on burgers, pizza, or the Zucchini Pasta (p. 243).

This sauce can either be served raw or simmered over low heat for about 10 minutes to further blend the flavors. If you choose to heat it, try stirring in 1/2 cup nutritional yeast for a cream-textured sauce.

1 cup sun-dried tomatoes
1 clove garlic
1 cup chopped tomatoes
1 cup water
1/2 cup grated cucumber

cont.

3 tbsp hemp oil

1 tbsp balsamic vinegar

1 tsp oregano

1 tsp rosemary

1/4 tsp thyme

Sea salt to taste

Soak the sun-dried tomatoes in the water for 20 minutes. Retain this water. In a food processor, process all ingredients, including sun-dried tomatoes water, until desired consistency is reached.

Keep refrigerated for up to 1 week.

Makes about 3 1/2 cups.

Sweet Pepper Hemp Pesto

raw option

This is a great burger topping. Full of flavor and nutrition, this pesto can also be used as a pizza sauce or even as a dip for crackers and vegetables.

2 cloves garlic

2 red bell peppers, cored and seeded

1/2 cup fresh basil

3 tbsp Nutritional Yeast and Sesame Seed Topping (p. 211)

2 tbsp hemp seeds

2 tbsp hemp oil

Sea salt to taste

In a food processor, process all ingredients together until smooth.

Keep refrigerated for up to 1 week.

Variation: Roast the peppers, lightly coated in coconut oil, for 30 minutes in a 300°F oven before blending. This will intensify the flavor.

Makes about 2 cups.

drinks

Quick and easy to make, these drinks are a good alternative to store-bought products.

Hemp Milk

raw

I usually make a week's supply of Hemp Milk at a time, which for me is about 8 cups. Hemp Milk is a good substitute for cow's milk on cereal. The chocolate version of this milk is also tasty on cereal, for variety. Hemp Milk also adds a smoothness and subtle flavor to smoothies.

- 3 1/2 cups water
- 1 cup hemp seeds
- 2 tbsp agave nectar

In blender, combine all ingredients.

Keep refrigerated for up to 2 weeks.

Makes about 4 cups.

Chocolate Hemp Milk

raw option

Use roasted carob powder if you like a fairly intense chocolate flavor. Use cacao nibs instead to make it raw chocolate milk. But be aware that raw cacao nibs also contain a small amount of caffeine.

- 3 1/2 cups water
- 1 cup hemp seeds
- 2 tbsp roasted carob powder (or 2 tbsp cacao nibs to make milk 100% raw)
- 2 tbsp agave nectar

In blender, combine all ingredients.

Keep refrigerated for up to 2 weeks.

Makes 4–4 1/2 cups.

Rooibos Almond Milk

This tasty, creamy mixture is delicious as a stand-alone drink or on cereal. Of course, it's packed with nutrition.

- 3 cups water
- 5 rooibos tea bags (or about 2 tbsp of loose rooibos if using a teaball)

cont.

1 cup soaked almonds
1 tbsp agave nectar
1 tbsp fresh lemon juice
Sea salt to taste

Bring 3 cups of water to a boil. Pour into a teapot; add rooibos. Let steep for 15 minutes. Remove teabags or teaball.

In blender, blend tea, almonds, agave nectar, lemon juice, and sea salt until smooth.

Keep refrigerated for up to 1 week.

Makes about 4 cups.

Ginger Ale

raw

This is a simple, healthful drink, especially refreshing in the summertime. The ginger froths up to give it an effervescent quality. Use sparkling mineral water in place of regular water if you want even more fizz. Because of the combination of raw lemon and ginger, this drink will help raise the body's pH and reduce inflammation.

1 lemon
2 cups water
1 tbsp agave nectar
1/2 tbsp grated fresh ginger
Sea salt to taste

Squeeze the juice of the lemon into a blender. Add water, agave nectar, ginger, and sea salt; blend.

Keep refrigerated for up to 2 weeks.

Makes about 2 cups.

desserts

I usually eat Vegetable Crackers (p. 259) or Zucchini Chips (p. 260) for dessert or as an evening snack; yet, every so often, I like to have a more traditional dessert. My Banana Coconut Pie is so nutritious that it can easily double as a healthy snack at any time of the day, and even as a post-exercise recovery food.

Banana Coconut Pie

raw

Full of complete protein, essential fatty acids, fiber, and many vitamins and minerals, the Banana Coconut Pie is much more than just a sweet snack. The pure, natural ingredients supply high nutrition in a traditional dessert form. Dinner guests love it.

Crust

1 cup fresh or soaked dried dates
1/2 cup shredded coconut
1/2 cup ground flaxseed
1/2 cup hemp flour
1/2 cup sunflower seeds
1 tbsp grated fresh ginger
1 tsp fresh lemon juice

Filling

2 bananas
1 pear
1/2 cup shredded coconut
1/2 cup macadamia nuts
1/4 cup hemp flour
1/4 cup sunflower seeds
1 tbsp grated fresh ginger
1/2 tsp salt

Topping

1/2 cup macadamia nuts
1/4 cup sunflower seeds
1/4 tsp cinnamon

Make crust by putting all ingredients in a food processor and processing until doughlike. Remove and spread out onto a pie plate; pack down.

Put all filling ingredients into food processor and process until creamy. Spread out evenly in pie crust.

Put topping ingredients into food processor; pulse a few times. Spread on top of pie filling.

Refrigerate until cool and firm, about 60 minutes.

Makes 8 servings.

appendix

vitamins and minerals

It's helpful to familiarize yourself with the various vitamins and minerals, understanding why they matter, what foods they are found in most plentifully, and, in turn, which Thrive Diet recipes are rich sources of each. Vitamins and minerals are an integral part of anyone's diet, regardless of activity level. However, many active people, and in particular competitive athletes, are often concerned that their diet does not supply enough nutrients. A program based on the principles of the Thrive Diet will provide all the nutrients needed for optimal health and peak athletic performance. The recipes I have created are a good source of all the nutrients a person needs to thrive: Fresh fruit, vegetables, pseudograins, legumes, nuts, and seeds are overwhelmingly present, providing healthy doses of vitamins and minerals.

vitamin A

Vitamin A helps the body resist infection, which it is more prone to after physical exertion, and allows the body to use its reserves for repairing and regenerating muscle tissue (instead of fighting infection)—leading to quicker recovery. Vitamin A helps support growth and repair of muscle and maintains red and white blood cells—crucial for performance.

Best Thrive sources: orange and dark green vegetables, including carrots, pumpkin, sweet potatoes, winter squash, broccoli, kale, parsley, and spinach; apricots, mango, papaya, cantaloupe.

vitamin B1

Vitamin B1 helps the body convert carbohydrate into energy. Maintaining high energy levels depends in part on maintaining adequate vitamin B1 in the diet. People who eat healthy rarely have a problem getting enough vitamin B1; it's plentiful in many foods. Also, because active people expend more energy than the average person, they need more vitamin B1. Again, this is usually not a problem, since with increased activity comes increased appetite.

Best Thrive sources: legumes, pseudograins, nuts, brown rice, nutritional yeast, and blackstrap molasses.

vitamin B2

Vitamin B2 helps break down amino acids (protein) for the body to use. Utilization of amino acids is a key factor in quick muscle recovery and regeneration after exertion. Like vitamin B1, B2 helps the body convert carbohydrate into energy.

Vitamin B2 aids in the formulation of growth hormones, a primary factor in muscle health and development. It also contributes to healthy red blood cell production. Red blood cells are the carriers of oxygen to working muscles, making them an integral part of performance.

Best Thrive sources: legumes, pseudograins, nuts, brown rice, nutritional yeast, and blackstrap molasses.

vitamin B3

Vitamin B3 is essential for the body's breakdown and utilization of carbohydrate and protein. As with other B vitamins, vitamin B3 plays

an integral part in the conversion of food into energy. Vitamin B3 has an important role in keeping the digestive system healthy as well. A healthy digestive system will allow the body to get more out of its food, reducing hunger and the amount of food needed. Also, a healthy digestive system will extract trace minerals from food, essential for performance.
Best Thrive sources: beets, sunflower seeds, nutritional yeast.

vitamin B5

As with other B vitamins, vitamin B5 helps the body convert food into energy. As well, vitamin B5 facilitates the production of steroids—an integral part of the regeneration process after exertion. This vitamin is found in a wide variety of healthy foods, and deficiency is uncommon.
Best Thrive sources: seeds, pseudograins, avocados.

vitamin B6

As a B vitamin, B6 too participates in the release of energy from food and in the formation of red blood cells. Vitamin B6 aids in the production of antibodies—essential for warding off infection and maintaining the ability to recover from exertion quickly. Vitamin B6 contributes to cardiovascular health, helping the heart efficiently circulate blood in a greater volume as demanded by the active person.
Best Thrive sources: pseudograins, bananas, brown rice, walnuts, avocados, oats.

vitamin B12

Vitamin B12 is essential for a healthy nervous system, aiding in coordination and smooth muscle movement. As with other B vitamins, B12 plays a role in the production of red blood cells and conversion of

food to usable energy. Unlike other B vitamins, B12 is not plentiful in foods. Special attention must be paid to ensure dietary B12 needs are met, particularly if the diet doesn't contain animal products and exercise level is moderate to high.
Best Thrive sources: chlorella, miso, nutritional yeast.

biotin

Biotin works in concert with the B vitamins as a converter of food into usable energy.
Best Thrive source: nuts, nutritional yeast.

vitamin C

Vitamin C is a powerful antioxidant, meaning it plays an integral role in reducing damage to body tissue and muscle done by physical activity; it is therefore essential for active people. Cellular damage that occurs as a result of environmental factors such as pollution will be minimized by daily ingestion of vitamin C. The ability to minimize environmental stress will greatly improve the body's ability to ward off infection and allow it to recover from physical activity considerably quicker. Iron absorption is improved when iron is ingested at the same time as vitamin C–rich foods.
Best Thrive sources: most vegetables and fruits (especially citrus fruits).

vitamin D

Vitamin D allows the body to absorb calcium more efficiently—a key factor for proper bone formation (and healing) and smooth muscle contractions.
Best Thrive sources: nutritional yeast, exposure to sunlight.

vitamin E

Vitamin E, like vitamin C, is a powerful antioxidant. Active people need higher levels of vitamin E than sedentary people, as vitamin E, in concert with others, reduces the constant stress exercise places on the body.

Promoting cardiovascular health by maintaining an optimal ratio of "good" to "bad" cholesterol is another role of vitamin E. The ability to maintain the ideal ratio is a key factor for proper growth hormone production—the cornerstone of muscle rejuvenation post-exertion. Vitamin E also combats the effects of harmful free radicals produced by physical activity.

Best Thrive sources: flaxseed oil, hemp oil, pumpkin seed oil, and especially raspberry seed, cranberry seed, and pomegranate seed oil; nuts, avocados.

vitamin K

Vitamin K plays a significant role in blood clotting. It also provides the heart with nutrients it needs for optimal function.

Best Thrive sources: leafy green vegetables, pine nuts.

folate (folic acid)

Folate is a B vitamin that is found naturally in foods; when in supplement form, it is called folic acid. Folate works in tandem with vitamin B12 to help produce oxygen-carrying red blood cells. Folate plays an integral role in helping the body make use of dietary protein, facilitating muscle repair. The heart relies on folate, in part, to help it maintain a smooth, rhythmic, efficient beat—and a higher tolerance for physical activity.

Best Thrive sources: leafy green vegetables, legumes, pseudograins, orange juice, nutritional yeast.

calcium

For most people, bone strength and repair is calcium's major role. Active people, however, have another important job for the mineral: muscle contraction and ensuring a rhythmic heat beat. Upward of 95 percent of the body's calcium is stored in the skeleton, and a decline in calcium levels may take years to manifest as osteoporosis. But a decline *will* be noticeable as an irregular heart beat and muscle cramps—the responsibilities of that remaining few percent. Since calcium in the bloodstream is lost in sweat and muscle contractions, a higher dietary level for active people is recommended.

The body orchestrates the effective combination of calcium and vitamin D to maximize calcium absorption.

Best Thrive sources: leafy green vegetables, unhulled sesame seeds, tahini.

chromium

Chromium works with other vitamins and minerals to turn carbohydrate into usable energy.

Best Thrive sources: pseudograins, nuts, nutritional yeast, black pepper, thyme.

copper

Like vitamin C, copper assists iron absorption in the body. With iron, copper plays a role in the transport of oxygen throughout the body—imperative for optimal performance. As a member of the body's defense network, copper works in concert with antioxidants to reduce effects of environmental and physical damage, providing the body with a strong platform to regenerate and build strength.

Best Thrive sources: legumes, seeds, pseudograins, raisins, nuts.

iodine

Iodine is integral to thyroid hormone production. Thyroid hormone assists the cells in the fabrication of protein and the metabolism of fats—essential for energy maintenance. High levels of iodine are lost in sweat, making active people's requirements higher than those of less active people.
Best Thrive sources: sea vegetables (especially dulse).

iron

The main role of iron is to fabricate hemoglobin to facilitate red blood cell health. An adequate iron level is of paramount importance for the active person. A well-maintained iron level ensures the body is able to deliver oxygen-rich blood to the hard-working extremities, maximizing efficacy. Also used to build blood proteins needed for food metabolism, digestion, and circulation, dietary iron is essential for proper functionality.
Best Thrive sources: spinach, legumes (especially split peas), pumpkin seeds.

magnesium

Critical for muscle function, magnesium helps the heart beat rhythmically by allowing it to relax between beats, which allows all other muscles to relax. Magnesium also assists in calcium's bone production.
Best Thrive sources: leafy green vegetables, string beans, legumes, pseudograins, bananas, nuts, avocados.

manganese

As an activator of antioxidant enzymes, manganese contributes to an expedited process of recovery, essential to all those who are physically

active. Manganese is a cofactor in energy production, metabolizing protein and fats.
Best Thrive sources: leafy green vegetables, legumes, pseudograins, nuts, brown rice.

molybdenum

A trace mineral, molybdenum's chief role is as a mobilizer, moving stored iron from the liver into the bloodstream—of particular significance to active people. An aid in the detoxification processes, molybdenum helps the body rid itself of potentially toxic material, minimizing stress.
Best Thrive sources: legumes, pseudograins, nuts.

phosphorus

Critical in the maintenance of the body's metabolic system, phosphorus allows the body to use food as fuel. Phosphorus works with calcium in the production, repair, and maintenance of bones.
Best Thrive sources: pseudograins, most tropical fruit.

potassium

Potassium, an electrolyte, helps the body maintain fluid balance and therefore hydration. Being properly hydrated is essential for efficient movement. Proper hydration will maintain the blood's light viscous flow, increasing the amount the heart can pump and improving performance. Smooth, concise muscle contractions are one of potassium's responsibilities. Nerve impulse transmission and cell integrity also rely, to a degree, on potassium. As a result, smooth motor function, heart beat efficiency, and the ability to strongly contract a muscle are dependent on adequate potassium intake. As

with other electrolytes, potassium is lost in sweat, so active people need more.
Best Thrive sources: leafy green vegetables, most fruits (especially bananas and kiwis).

selenium

In concert with vitamin E, selenium preserves muscle tissue elasticity, allowing fluent, supple movement. A trace mineral, selenium combines with other antioxidants to shield red blood cells from damage done by physical exertion. It also improves immune function. As with other antioxidants, selenium offers protection from environmental stress encountered by most people on a regular basis.
Best Thrive sources: Brazil nuts, walnuts, brown rice, nutritional yeast.

zinc

Zinc's major role is to allow the body to use dietary protein as building blocks, for the regeneration of muscles. As well, zinc plays an integral role in the preservation of proper immune function.
Best Thrive sources: pseudograins, pumpkin seeds, nutritional yeast.

carbohydrate, fat, and protein

carbohydrate

Carbohydrate is abundant, present in most foods to at least some degree. For nonactive people, a regular diet will supply the body with all the carbohydrate it needs. For active people, however, increased dietary carbohydrate is essential for maintaining energy levels and replenishing muscles post-exertion. Carbohydrate also assists in the digestion and utilization of all other foods.

Carbohydrates are made up of three components: sugar, starch, and fiber. When grains are refined, the fiber is removed, increasing the percentage of starch and sugar. These are the "bad" carbohydrates. Unfortunately, they are the ones most plentiful in the typical North American diet of refined carbohydrates. White bread, pasta, donuts, and other such foods make up the vast majority of the average North American's carbohydrate intake. Fiber-rich whole grains and fruit in particular, on the other hand, are "good" carbohydrate, needed by the body in order to be healthy and function optimally. And as you know, optimal health leads to optimal, lean body composition. In addition, refined, processed carbohydrates cause inflammation to develop in the body. Inflammation is the precursor to visible signs of premature aging. In contrast, carbohydrate derived from raw fruit helps reduce inflammation, contributing to quicker recovery from exercise and slowing of biological aging.

The first symptoms exhibited by people who limit healthy carbohydrates for a prolonged period are mental lethargy and increased general fatigue. If a carbohydrate-restrictive diet is maintained for an extended period, it can lead to internal organ damage and, ironically, a reduction in lean muscle and the accumulation of excess body fat. Complex carbohydrates derived from whole grains are an excellent source of fuel for the muscles and brain.

Best Thrive sources: vegetables, pseudograins, fruit.

fat

When the body is engaged in a low-intensity activity, fat is its primary source of energy. (Carbohydrate takes over once intensity increases.) Fat ensures that fat-soluble vitamins A, D, E, and K are delivered and utilized in the body. Fat-soluble vitamins play a major role in overall health; dietary fat helps activate and transport them.

Best Thrive sources: flaxseed, hemp, and pumpkin in seed and oil form; avocado.

Essential Fatty Acids Omega-3 and omega-6 are the two essential fatty acids (EFAs), *essential* meaning that the body cannot produce them—they must be ingested, by eating foods rich in EFA. EFAs are a type of fat known as long-chain polyunsaturated fatty acids.

EFAs are an important dietary component of overall health. Lending support to the healthy function of the cardiovascular, immune, and nervous systems, EFAs also play an integral role in promoting cell health. Repair and regeneration of the cellular membrane is vital for keeping the body biologically young and enabling it to retain mobility and vitality throughout life. Contributing to our cells' ability to receive nutrition and eliminate waste, EFAs help keep the cellular regeneration process moving. Our body's ability to fight off infection and reduce inflammation is in part dependent on having an adequate supply of EFAs in the diet. Healthy and efficient brain development in children has been linked to a diet rich in EFAs.

A balance of omega-3 and omega-6 EFAs is vital for skin health. Dry skin is commonly treated topically with a moisturizer, leaving the cause of the problem unaddressed. A diet with adequate EFAs will keep skin looking and feeling supple.

Best Thrive sources: omega-3: flaxseed, flaxseed oil, all hemp products (protein, flour, seed, oil), walnuts; omega-6: hemp products (protein, flour, seed, oil), seeds, most nuts, vegetable oils (including extra-virgin olive oil), avocados.

protein

Protein assists in the fabrication of hormones, enzymes, and antibodies. Well-formed hormones are essential for a vast number of functions; muscle repair and preservation during exertion are just two. One task of enzymes is to extract nutrients from food so that the body is able to make use of them. Shielding the body from bacteria and viral infection (such as the common cold) are the responsibility of antibodies, which are formulated once dietary protein is ingested. Protein is most praised for its ability to supply broken-down muscles with the building blocks needed to rebuild even stronger. Combined with carbohydrate, protein is able to infuse a tired muscle with more energy than carbohydrate could by itself.

Best sources: leafy green vegetables, legumes, pseudograins, seeds (especially hemp).

glossary

Ancient grains Ancient grains are those that have not been altered over time by either primitive crossing techniques or modern genetic modification. Spelt, barley, teff, and millet are all ancient grains.

Antioxidants "Antioxidants" is the name given to several naturally occurring compounds, including vitamins C and E and the mineral selenium. Carotenoids, the compound responsible for the different colors of vegetables, act as antioxidants. Antioxidants are most prized for their ability to protect cells. Helping rid the body of free radicals, antioxidants are credited with helping maintain cellular health and regeneration. If not for antioxidants, cellular damage caused by several kinds of stress would advance quickly and possibly lead to cancer and other diseases.
Best Thrive sources: colorful vegetables, berries, cold-pressed oils.

Biological age Biological age refers to the time that has passed since the body's most recent round of cellular regeneration. Biological age can be reduced by speeding the regeneration process of the body. Complementary stress such as exercise and high-quality food reduces biologically age, while uncomplementary stress and refined foods increase it.

Biological debt Biological debt refers to the state of fatigue the body goes into after energy from stimulation has dissipated. It is often brought about by eating refined sugar or drinking coffee to gain short-term energy.

Celiac disease Celiac disease is the intolerance of gluten-containing foods, such as wheat. A celiac who consumes gluten risks damaging the small intestine.

Electrolytes Electrolytes are salts with electricity conductive properties. Throughout our body tissue, fluid, and blood, electrolytes conduct charges that are essential for muscle contractions, heart beats, fluid regulation, and general nerve function. Chloride, calcium, magnesium, sodium, and potassium are the chief minerals in electrolytes. A diet too low in these minerals can cause muscle cramps and heart palpitations. When too much fluid that does not contain electrolytes is drunk, it can flush out the body's remaining electrolytes, causing muscle cramping and heart palpitations.

People who lose electrolytes through means other than exercise are best replenishing their levels by means other than sport drinks, since these drinks also supply unwanted sugar. Diarrhea, vomiting, and other losses in bodily fluid will require electrolyte replenishment. Eating dulse is a good way to replenish them.
Best Thrive sources: seaweed (especially dulse), citrus fruit, sport drinks (recipes begin on page 122).

Empty food Sometimes referred to as empty calories, this term is usually assigned to foods that are heavily processed or refined. With little if any nutritional value, such foods still retain their calories and usually starch and sugar, which can lead to quick weight gain and a feeling of never being satisfied.

Essential fatty acids See Appendix, page 283.

Fatty acids The difference between fatty acids and essential fatty acids is that the body is able to produce fatty acids, while essential fatty acids must come from food sources. (See Essential Fatty Acids in Appendix, page 283.)

Free radicals Damaging compounds that alter cell membranes and can adversely affect our DNA, free radicals are not something we want too many of. Occurring naturally in the body, free radicals are produced on a daily basis in small amounts. However, as stress increases, so too does the production of free radicals. If stress is allowed to persist in the body for an extended period, the damage done by free radicals can be significant; it has been linked to cancer and other serious diseases. Free radicals have also been shown to cause premature signs of aging when allowed to remain in the system. A reduction of stress through better nutrition is one way to combat free radical production. Specifically, antioxidants help rid the body of free radicals, by helping it excrete them in urine and sweat.

Fructose Also known as fruit sugar, fructose is naturally occurring in most fruits. Since it is very sweet, it is often extracted from fruits to sweeten other foods.

Glucose Glucose is a form of simple carbohydrate and is the primary sugar found in the blood.
Best Thrive source: dates.

Lignans Lignans are plant-derived compounds that combine with others to fabricate the cell wall of the plant. Lignans are regarded as one of the best compounds to help protect against cancer and reduce cholesterol levels. Upon consumption of lignan-rich foods, friendly bacteria convert lignans to mammalian lignan, releasing their therapeutic attributes in the body.
Best Thrive sources: flaxseeds, pumpkin seeds, sesame seeds.

Net gain Net gain is the term I use to refer to the usable nutrition the body is left with once food is digested and assimilated. The more the body must work to digest food, the more energy will be lost, mostly to heat, sometimes leaving the body with a net loss.

Nutrient dense Also referred to as nutrient-rich, nutrient-dense foods are those that are unrefined and, as such, packed with nutrition. Some foods are inherently more nutrient dense than others; those with high levels of antioxidants and an abundance of vitamins and minerals are said to be nutrient dense.

One-step nutrition One-step nutrition is a term I have assigned to foods that contain a form of nutrients that can be directly used by the body, without having to be broken down first. For example, simple carbohydrate found in fruit can be directly used by the body for energy, with a high rate of efficiency. Amino acids and essential fatty acids are other examples of one-step nutrition. Each time nutrients are altered by the body so that it can make use of them, energy is lost.

Phytonutrient Also referred to as a phytochemical, a phytonutrient is a plant compound that, by boosting the immune system, offers health benefits independent of merely its nutritional value. Classified as a micronutrient, phytonutrients are not essential for life, but they can help improve vitality and, in turn, quality of life.
Best Thrive sources: vegetables, seeds, fruit, nuts, green tea, yerba maté, rooibos.

Primary-source foods Crops that have been grown for direct consumption are primary-source foods. Animals that are raised for food or for their products, such as milk or eggs, are secondary-source foods. They consume primary-source foods, and then humans eat them. An extra step is added when secondary rather than primary foods are consumed, requiring more energy to be used and lost.

Probiotic Probiotic is a Greek word meaning "for life." Known as "good" bacteria, probiotics support beneficial intestinal flora. Maintaining good intestinal flora will help the body digest, process, and utilize complex carbohydrates and protein. The regular consumption of probiotics increases the bioavailability of minerals, especially calcium.

Recalibrate The altering of one or more of the body's senses, recalibration is required when trying to reduce the amount of stimuli needed to gain energy. It is used to change the body's "perception" of food. When stimulating food is eliminated from the diet, the body will be able to gain energy from natural, whole foods and therefore have no need for unhealthy stimulating foods.

Simple carbohydrate Also known as simple sugar, simple carbohydrate is prevalent in most fruits. The body's most usable and therefore first choice for fuel, simple carbohydrate is necessary for both mental and physical activity. If the body is not fed foods that contain simple carbohydrate, it will have to convert complex carbohydrates, but that takes extra work and so is not a good use of energy.

Glucose and fructose, the primary components of simple carbohydrate, are the best fuel in that they are already in a form the body can utilize. Plus, digestive enzymes are able to break them down more efficiently than they can complex carbohydrate.
Best Thrive sources: fruit of all kinds.

Sterols Sterols are steroid-like compounds found in both plants and animals. Plant sterols have the ability to lower cholesterol and have been recognized as beneficial to heart health and in the fight against cardiovascular disease. All the major sources of plant sterols are plentiful in the Thrive Diet.
Best Thrive sources: vegetables, legumes, fruit, nuts, seeds, and seed oils, particularly hemp, flaxseed, and pumpkin.

Trace minerals Also known as microminerals, trace minerals have several important functions in the body that add up to optimal health.

As the name suggests, these minerals are needed only in trace amounts, and a diet rich in a variety of foods will ensure their inclusion.
Best Thrive sources: most foods to some degree, but especially seaweed, yerba maté, maca, green tea.

Trans fats Also known as trans-fatty acids, these are a form of fat produced by heating oils to high temperature, thus altering their chemical compound and making these fats difficult for the body to process. They also inhibit the body's ability to efficiently burn healthy fats as fuel.

Whole foods Foods that have not had any part removed during processing are known as whole foods. The term *whole food* is also used to refer to foods that are simply in their natural state, such as fresh raw fruit and vegetables.

resources

THRIVEDIET
Approved
This quality product meets the nutritional standards as outlined in my book.
Brendan Brazier, bestselling author
www.thrivediet.com

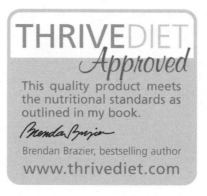

When shopping for products, you can be assured that the ones bearing this logo meet the highest nutritional standards as outlined in this book. The following list contains foods that I've personally tested and use myself—they are *Thrive Diet Approved*.

Vega: plant-based whole-food products

I formulated *Vega Whole Food Health Optimizer* to replicate the smoothie that I first made for myself at the age of 15 to help speed recovery after exercise—a meal and all my supplements in liquid form. It supplies complete protein, essential fatty acids, probiotics, fiber, enzymes, antioxidants, chlorella, and maca, while maintaining a slightly alkaline pH level in the body. *Vega Whole Food Health Optimizer* (formerly called Vega Whole Food Meal Replacement) is a whole-food powder that can be mixed with water to supply complete nutrition anytime, anywhere.

Vega Whole Food Energy Bars were the next creation in the Vega line. These are 100 percent raw bars, based on the recipe that I've been making in a food processor for years. Moist, fresh, and enzyme-rich, these bars are indispensable on a long bicycle ride or when you know you're going to miss a meal. They include sprouted flax, sprouted mung bean, agave nectar, and wheat grass.

Vega Whole Food Smoothie Infusion is a simplified version of the *Vega Whole Food Health Optimizer,* containing many of the same basic ingredients but without the food-source vitamins and minerals. It's a neutral-tasting whole-food powder that gives a convenient, instant boost of complete protein, omega-3, fiber, and greens to any smoothie. It can be used in place of hemp protein and flax in all smoothie recipes in this book to make them even more nutrient dense and alkaline forming. It can also serve as a more nutritionally complete replacement for hemp protein and flax in all Thrive Diet baking recipes on a 1:1 ratio. Additionally, up to 20 percent of regular flour can be substituted for Vega Whole Food Smoothie Infusion in traditional recipes.

Vega Antioxidant EFA Oil Blend is a synergistic, balanced blend of unrefined, cold-pressed plant-based oils rich in omega-3 and omega-6 essential fatty acids. In addition to the hemp, flax, and pumpkin seed oils, I added a synergistic combination of antioxidant oils to reduce cellular oxidization and inflammation. They are: green tea seed, pomegranate seed, black cumin seed, black raspberry seed, blueberry seed, and cranberry seed. I also added coconut oil for its MTC content.

Vega products are made by Sequel Naturals and available at most health food stores, some grocery stores, and online.

Tel: 1-866-839-8863
Email: info@sequelnaturals.com
www.myvega.com

Guayaki: yerba maté

Guayaki yerba maté is shade-grown under the natural jungle canopy, thereby shielding its leaves from direct sunlight, keeping them subtle. Unlike some yerba maté that is produced in plantation-style farms, Guayaki is grown with the jungle, not instead of the jungle. This type of agriculture helps preserve the natural ecosystem and is good for local farmers because they can make more money by selling maté than they could by clearing the land to graze cattle. I use Guayaki yerba maté in several of my recipes; it's particularly good in the exercise-specific ones. Available in most health food stores and online.

Tel: 1-888-482-9254
Email: info@guayaki.com
www.guayaki.com

Aviva Yerba mate is also an excellent choice and can be ordered online:
Tel: 1-877-255-1473
Email: contact@yerba-mate.com
www.yerba-mate.com

Maine Coast: sea vegetables

With a focus on sustainability, Maine Coast hand harvests wild organic sea vegetables off the coast of Maine. I use many of its seaweeds in my recipes because they are premium quality and free of toxins. The company's wide variety of sea vegetables is available in most health food stores, many grocery stores, and online.

Tel: 207-565-2907
Email: info@seaveg.com
www.seaveg.com

Manitoba Harvest: hemp

Manitoba Harvest grows premium-quality hemp, turning it into hemp food in the form of raw protein powder, hemp seed, cold-pressed oil, and flour, all also top quality. Never using herbicides or pesticides on its products, Manitoba Harvest is a first-rate model of sustainable agriculture. The company uses a low-temperature milling process that preserves all the natural goodness of the plant, further increasing its food value. Available in most health food stores, many grocery stores, and online.

Tel: 1-800-665-4367
Email: info@manitobaharvest.com
www.manitobaharvest.com

NOW: cold pressed oils, rooibos, stevia

NOW makes high-quality, cold-pressed, raw organic oils. All its oils are obtained from the first pressing, and solvents are never used in the extraction process. The oils include coconut, macadamia, flaxseed, extra-virgin olive, grape seed, and avocado. I use cold-pressed coconut oil and flaxseed oil in several of my recipes. NOW also manufactures high-quality organic rooibos tea and stevia. NOW products are available in most health food stores.

Tel: 1-800-283-3500
www.nowfoods.com

O.N.E.: coconut water

O.N.E. is 100 percent natural coconut water with no preservatives. It's naturally filtered for nine months through the fibers of the coconut, creating a pure isotonic beverage—a convenient and practical alternative to hacking open fresh young coconuts with a machete. O.N.E coconut water is bottled at the source in Brazil; therefore, the rest of the coconut doesn't need to be transported, which saves energy. In addition, most whole young coconuts transported to North America are dipped in formaldehyde as a preservative. In many cases, traces of formaldehyde are detectable in the water and meat, so O.N.E is a healthier alternative. I use O.N.E. as the base of my sport drinks and in several other recipes. Available in most heath food stores and some grocery stores.

Tel: 1-888-663-2626
Email: info@onecoco.com
www.onecoco.com

Organics Unlimited: bananas, plantains

Organically grown on carefully cared for farms in nutrient-rich soil, Organics Unlimited bananas and plantains are of premium quality. The GROW (Giving Resources and Opportunities to Workers) Foundation, a nonprofit organization dedicated to helping farm laborers make better lives for themselves and their families, was founded by Organics Unlimited. Organics Unlimited bananas and plantains are available in some health food stores and select grocery stores.

Tel: 619-710-0658
Email: info@organicsunlimited.com
www.organicsunlimited.com

Salba: white chia

Salba white chia is the most nutritionally dense form of chia available. Salba white chia is grown in the extremely nutrient-rich soil surrounding the Amazon Basin in Peru, where it flourishes. Salba white chia has a higher percentage of both protein and omega-3 than standard chia. I add salba to many of my salads. Available in health food stores.

Tel: 1-877-337-2522
Email: info@sourcesalba.com
www.sourcesalba.com

Sambazon: açaí
Importers of high-quality açaí berries from Brazil, Sambazon packs them within two days of their harvest to maintain top nutrient value. They are then frozen or freeze dried and shipped to the United States so that their nutrition value stays at its peak. Sambazon helps preserve the Amazon Rainforest by paying small family farmers fair wages, thereby making it more lucrative for the locals to harvest açaí than to sell the trees for lumber.

Tel: 877-726-2296
Email: info@sambazon.com
www.sambazon.com

Sequel Naturals: maca, chlorella
Along with my Vega products, Sequel Naturals produces MacaSure and ChlorEssence, both of which are used in my Vega formulation.

MacaSure is made from 100 percent organic maca root, grown traditionally in nutrient-rich volcanic soil of the high Andean highlands of Peru. The gelatinization process used to remove the starch from the maca concentrates the active ingredients and improves the maca's absorption once in the body. Gelatinization does not involve the use of gelatin.

ChlorEssence brand chlorella contains the highest CGF concentration of any brand of chlorella, with values ranging from 18 to 25 percent. ChlorEssence is grown outdoors in rich, spring-fed freshwater ponds on subtropical Japanese coral islands. Unlike some chemically cracked cell chlorella, ChlorEssence cell walls are jet-sprayed to achieve over 80 percent digestibility without compromising potency or shelf life. Available in most health food stores, some grocery stores, and online.

Tel: 1-866-839-8863
Email: info@sequelnaturals.com
www.sequelnaturals.com

Stahlbush Island Farms: frozen fruits and vegetables

Stahlbush Island Farms grows, harvests, and freezes premium-quality, ready-to-eat fruits and vegetables without adding sugar or preservatives. I often use this company's fruit when making my daily smoothie. It's a fast and convenient way to add high-quality fruit to your diet. Located in Oregon, Stahlbush Island Farms adheres to sustainable farming practices, including crop rotation. This practice benefits not only the nutrient value of their produce, but also helps preserve agricultural and environmental health. Available in most health food stores.

Tel: 541-757-1497
Email: sif@stahlbush.com
www.stahlbush.com

Touch Organic: green and white tea

Touch Organic's green tea series consist of high-quality organic tea blends that are produced at the source in southeastern China. I use these teas in several of my recipes to infuse the food with flavor and extra nutrition. They can be found in major grocery, health, pharmacy, and specialty stores.

Tel: 250-837-4655
Email: info@graham.com.hk
www.touchorganic.com

Vita-Mix: Blender

The use of a Vita-Mix machine is the best way to maintain the natural state of food and, at the same time, improve the bioavailability of nutrients by liquefying. I use a Vita-Mix when making many of my recipes including soups, sauces, smoothies and energy gels. This machine features a powerful motor, top quality materials and workmanship, and it is designed to last. Its sharp, stainless-steel blades easily cut through all kinds of vegetables—even harder ones such as carrots. The Vita-Mix is the most versatile and most reliable kitchen appliance I have. Available online.

Tel: 800-848-2649
Email: household@vitamix.com
www.vitamix.com

Recommended Reading

Books

Eat To Live
Joel Fuhrman
www.drfuhrman.com

The China Study
T. Colin Campbell, Thomas M. Campbell II
www.thechinastudy.com

Web Sites

G Living Network
The modern green lifestyle network dedicated to environmental preservation, with style.
www.gliving.com

Nutrition MD
Helping people adopt healthier diets
www.nutritionmd.org

references

Adlercreutz, H. Western diet and Western diseases: Some hormonal and biochemical mechanisms and associations. *Scand J Clin Lab Invest* 1990, 201 (Suppl):3S–23S.

Alfino, Mark, John S. Caputo, and Robin Wynyard, eds. *McDonaldization Revisited: Critical Essay on Consumer Culture.* Westport, CT: Praeger, 1998.

Bravo, L. Polyphenols: Chemistry, dietary sources, metabolism, and nutritional significance. *Nutr Rev* 1998, 56(2):317–33.

Burke, E.R. *Optimal Muscle Recovery.* New York: Avery Publishing Group, 1999.

Campbell, C.J. *The Coming Oil Crisis.* Essex, UK: Multi-Science and Petroconsultants, 1997.

Cao, G., et al. Antioxidant capacity of tea and common vegetables. *J Agric Food Chem* 1996, 44:3426–31.

———. Increases in human plasma antioxidant capacity after consumption of controlled diets high in fruit and vegetables. *Am J Clin Nutr* 1998, 68:1081–87.

Colgan, M. *Essential Fats.* Vancouver: Apple Publishing, 1998.

———. *Hormonal Health.* Vancouver: Apple Publishing, 1995.

———. *Optimum Sports Nutrition.* New York: Advanced Research Press, 1993.

———. *Protein for Muscle and Strength.* Vancouver: Apple Publishing, 1998.

———. *The New Nutrition.* Vancouver: Apple Publishing, 1996.

Conrad, C. *Hemp for Health: The Medicinal and Nutritional Uses of Cannabis Sativa.* Rochester, VT: Inner Traditions International, 1997.

Consumers Union Education Services. *Captive Kids: A Report on Commercial Pressures on Kids at School.* Yonkers, NY: Consumers Union, 1998.

Cordain, L. *The Paleo Diet: Lose Weight and Get Healthy by Eating the Food You Were Designed to Eat.* New York: John Wiley and Son, 2001.

Coulstron, A.M. The role of dietary fats in plant-based diets. *Am J Clin Nutr* 1999, 70 (Suppl):512S–15S.

Coyne, L.L. *Fat Won't Make You Fat*. Calgary, AB: Fish Creek Publishing, 1998.

De Kloet, E.R. Corticosteroids, stress, and aging. *Annals of New York Academy of Sciences* 1992, 663:358.

Erasmus, U. *Fats and Oils*. Vancouver: Alive Books, 1986.

Fabris, N., et al., eds. *Physiopathological Processes of Aging*. New York: Academy of Sciences, 1992.

Ferrandiz, M.L., et al. Anti-inflammatory activity and inhibition of arachidonic acid metabolism by flavonoids. *Agents Actions* 1991, 32:283–88.

Gabor, Maté. *When the Body Says No: The Cost of Hidden Stress*. Toronto: Vintage Canada, 2004.

Giese, A.C. *Living with Our Sun's Ultraviolet Rays*. Plenum Press, 1976.

Graci, S. *The Power of Super Foods: 30 Days That Will Change Your Life*. Toronto: Prentice Hall Canada, 1997.

Green, M.B. *Eating Oil: Energy Use in Food Production*. Boulder, CO: Westview Press, 1978.

Hall, J.V. Valuing the health benefits of clean air. *Science* 1992, 255:812–16.

Hart, A. *Adrenaline and Stress: The Exciting New Breakthrough That Helps You Overcome Stress Damage*. Rev. ed. Waco, TX: Word Publishing, 1995.

Hayflick, L. *How and Why We Age*. New York: Ballantine, 1994.

Holick, M.F. Vitamin D: The underappreciated D-lightful hormone that is important for skeletal and cellular health. *Curr Opin Endocrinal Diabetes* 2002, 9:87–98.

Howell E., and M. Murray. *Enzyme Nutrition*. Twin Lakes, WI: Lotus Press, 1986.

Hunter, Beatrice T. *The Natural Foods Primer*. New York: Simon and Schuster, 1972.

Joseph, J.A., et al. Oxidative stress production and vulnerability in aging: Putative nutritional implications for intervention. *Mech Ageing Dev* 2000, 116(2–3):141–53.

Kikuzaki, H., Y. Kawasaki, and N. Nakatani. Structure of antioxidative compounds in ginger. *ACS Symposium Series* 1994, 547:237–43.

King, B.J. *Fat Wars Action Planner*. Toronto: John Wiley and Sons, 2003.

King, B.J., and M.A. Schmidt. *Bio-Age: Ten Steps to a Younger You*. Toronto: Macmillan Canada, 2001.

Kraemer, W.J., et al. Effects of heavy-resistance training on hormonal response patterns in younger and older men. *J Appl Physiol* 1999, 87(3):982–92.

Krebs-Smith, S.M., et al. The effects of variety in food choices on dietary quality. *J Am Diet Assoc* 1987, 87(7):896–903.

Kushi, M., and A. Kushi. *Macrobiotic Diet*. New York: Japan Publication, 1985.

Kusnecov, A., and B.S. Rabin. Stressor-induced alterations of immune function: Mechanisms and issues. *Int Arch Allergy Immunol* 1994, 105(2):108.

Ley, B.M. *Maca: Adaptogen and Hormonal Regulator*. Detroit Lakes, MN: BL Publications, 2003.

———. *Chlorella: The Ultimate Green Food*. Detroit Lakes, MN: BL Publications, 2003.

Lardinois, C.K. The role of omega-3 fatty acids on insulin secretion and insulin sensitivity. *Med Hypotheses* 1997, 24(3): 243–48.

Leibowitz, S., et al. Insulin plays role in controlling fat craving. New York: News from the Rockefeller University, 1995.

Levenstein, Harvey. *Paradox of Plenty: A Social History of Eating in Modern America*. New York: Oxford University Press, 1993.

Levine, S., and H. Ursin. What Is Stress? In *Psychobiology of Stress,* ed. S. Levine and H. Ursin, 17. New York: Academic Press.

Loche, S.E. Stress, adaptation, and immunity: Studies in humans. *General Hospital Psychiatry* 1982, 4:49–58.

McCormick, D.B., D. Bier, and R.J. Cousins, eds. *Annual Review of Nutrition,* vol. 22. Palo Alto, CA: Annual Reviews, 2002.

McNeal, James U. *Kids as Consumers: A Handbook of Marketing to Children*. New York: Lexington Books, 1992.

Messina, M. Legumes and soybeans: Overview of their nutritional profiles and health effects. *Am J Clin Nutr* 1999, 70(3) (Suppl):439S–50S.

Nattrass, Brian, and Mary Altomare. *The Natural Step for Business: Wealth, Ecology and the Environmental Corporation*. Gabriola Island, BC: New Society, 2001.

Nick, G.L. Detoxification properties of low-dose phytochemical complexes found within select vegetables. *JANA* 2002, 5(4):34–44.

Nuernberger, P. *Freedom from Stress*. Honesdale, PA: Himalayan International Institute, 1981.

Perricone, N. *The Wrinkle Cure: Unlock the Power of Cosmeceuticals for Supple, Youthful Skin*. New York: Warner Books, 2001.

Pert C. *Molecules of Emotions: Why You Feel the Way You Feel*. New York: Touchstone, 1999, 22–23.

Pieri C., et al. Melatonin as an effective antioxidant. *Arch Gerontol Geriatr* 1995, 20:159–65.

Pollan, Michael. *Omnivore's Dilemma: A Natural History of Four Meals*. New York: Penguin, 2006.

Prasad, C. Food, mood and health: A neurobiologic outlook. *Braz J Med Biol Res* 1998, 31(12):1517–27.

Quillin, P. *Beating Cancer with Nutrition*. Tulsa, OK: Nutrition Times Press, 1994.

Rankin, J.W. Role of protein in exercise. *Clin Sports Med* 1999, 18(3):499–511.

Reiter, R.J. Oxygen radical detoxification processes during aging: The functional importance of melatonin. *Aging Clin Exp Res* 1995, 7:340–51.

Richardson J.H., T. Palmenton, and H. Chenan. The effect of calcium on muscle fatigue. *J Sports Med* 1980, 20:149.

Robinson, R. *The Hemp Manifesto: 101 Ways That Hemp Can Save Our World*. Rochester, VT: Inner Traditions International, 1997.

Sacks, Oliver. *The Man Who Mistook His Wife for a Hat and Other Clinical Tales*. New York: HarperPerennial, 1990.

Schmidt, M.A. *Smart Fats*. Berkeley, CA: North Atlantic Books, 1997.

Sears, B. *The Anti-Aging Zone*. New York: HarperCollins, 1999.

Seeman, T.E., and B.S. McEwen. Impact of social environmental characteristics on neuroendocrine regulation. *Psychosomatic Medicine* 1996, 58:462.

Simopoulos, A.P. Essential fatty acids in health and chronic disease. *Am J Clin Nutr* 1990, 70 (Suppl):560S–69S.

Somer, E., and N.L. Snyderman. *Food and Mood: The Complete Guide to Eating Well and Feeling Your Best*. New York: Owl Books, 1999.

Stanitski, C. Air pollution affects exercise performance. *Clin Sports Med* 1986, 4:725–26.

Stoll, A.L. *The Omega 3 Connection*. New York: Simon and Schuster, 2001.

Teitelbaum, J.E., and W.A. Walker. Nutritional impact of pre- and probiotics as protective gastrointestinal organisms. *Annu Rev Nutr* 2002, 22:107–38.

Van Cauter, E., and G. Copinschi. Interrelationships between growth hormone and sleep. *Growth Horm IGH Res* 10 (Suppl B) 2000:57S–62S.

Vandler, A.J. *Nutritional Stress and Toxic Chemicals*. Ann Arbor: University of Michigan Press, 1981.

Viru, A. *Hormones in Muscular Activity*. Boca Raton, FL: CRC Press, 1985.

Wilson, J.L. *Adrenal Fatigue: The 21st-Century Stress Syndrome*. Petaluma, CA: Smart Publications, 2002.

Wood, R. *The New Whole Foods Encyclopedia: A Comprehensive Resource for Healthy Eating*. New York: Penguin, 1999.

Wright, S. Essential fatty acids and the skin. *Br J Derm* 1991, 125:503–15.

Wurtman, J.J., and S. Suffers. *The Serotonin Solution*. New York: Ballantine Books, 1997.

Youdim, K.A., A. Martin, and J.A. Joseph. Essential fatty acids and the brain: Possible health implications. *Int J Dev Neurosci* 2000, 18:383–99.

Young. V.R., and P.L. Pellett. Plant proteins in relation to human protein and amino acid nutrition. *Am J Clin Nutr* 1994, 59 (5 Suppl):1203S–12S.

recipe index

Adzuki Bean Quinoa Sesame Pizza, 237
Almond Flaxseed Burger, 233
Apple Cinnamon Energy Bars, 229
Arame Seaweed Salad, 251
Avocado Cayenne Salad, 248

Balsamic Vinaigrette, 256
Banana Bread Energy Bars, 230
Banana Chocolate Pancakes, 214
Banana Coconut Pie, 270–271
Banana Ginger Pear Cereal, 215–216
Basic Electrolyte Sport Drink, 122
beverages, 127–128, 267–269
Black Bean Lime Salsa, 264–265
Black-Eyed Pea Cayenne Salsa, 265
Blood Builder Smoothie, 224
Blueberry Pancakes, 213
Blueberry Rooibos Antioxidant Smoothie, 224
Buckwheat Pancakes, 212
burgers, 232–233

Caesar Dressing, 255–256
Carob Gel, 124
Cayenne Dill Tahini Dressing, 253
cereals, 215–217
Chickpea Curry Pizza, 236
Chili Kidney Bean Pizza, 238–239
Chocolate Almond Smoothie, 223
Chocolate Blueberry Energy Bars, 228
Chocolate Hemp Milk, 268
Citrus Papaya Yerba Maté Energy Bars, 231–232
Coconut Carob Gel (with protein), 124–125
crackers, 257–261
Creamy Carrot Salad, 250
Creamy Ginger Carrot Soup, 245
Creamy Ginger Dressing, 254
Creamy Nutritional Yeast Sauce, 262
Creamy Pepper Soup, 246
Crunchy Cinnamon Plantain and Macadamia Nut Salad, 248–249
Crunchy Cinnamon Plantain Strips, 242–243
Cucumber Dill Dressing, 256–257
Cucumber Dill Salad, 249
Cucumber Pesto Salad, 250–251
Curry Lentil Crackers, 259
Curry Lentil Rice Pizza, 239
Curry Powder, 210

desserts, 269–271
Dinosaur Kale Quinoa Wrap, 241–242
dips, 261–267
Direct Fuel Bites, 125
dressings, 251–257
drinks, 127–129, 267–269

EFA Oil Blend, 210
Electrolyte Sport Drink with Ginger, 122
energy bars, 226–232
Energy Pudding, 125–126
exercise-specific recipes, 122–129

fast fuel, 123–125

Garlic Oregano Yam Oven Fries, 244
Ginger Ale, 269
Ginger Carrot Dressing, 254–255
Ginger Lime Squash, 241
Ginger Papaya Recovery, 127–128
Ginger Pear Energy Bars, 228–229
Ginger Pear Smoothie, 223
green smoothies, 225–226
Green Soup, 246
Green Tea Ginger Lime Crackers, 258–259
Green Tea Miso Gravy, 264

Hemp Milk, 268

Kale Calcium Boost Smoothie, 226
Ketchup, 261–262
kid-friendly recipes, 75–76

Lemon Crisp Beet Salad, 249–250
Lemon Ginger Plantain with Dulse, 242
Lemon-Lime Gel, 124
Lemon-Lime Recovery Drink, 127
Lemon-Lime Sport Drink, 123
Lemon Rooibos Crackers, 258
Lemon Sesame Crisps, 260–261

Macadamia Dill Dressing, 255
Mango Chutney, 263
Mango Coconut Energy Bars, 231
Mango Lime Dressing, 254
Mango Lime Hot Pepper Smoothie, 225
Mint Carob Sport Drink, 122–123
Miso Kelp Guacamole, 263–264

Nutritional Yeast and Sesame Seed Topping, 211

Orange Pumpkin Seed Dressing, 255

pancakes, 128–129, 211–215
Pecan Sunflower Burger, 233
Performance Banana Pancakes, 128–129
Pineapple Salsa, 265–266
pizza sauce, 235
pizzas, 234–240
Pomegranate Amaranth Energy Bars, 230–231
Pomegranate Green Tea Pancakes, 213–214
Pomegranate Poppy Seed Dressing, 257
Pomegrante Smoothie, 225
Popped Amaranth, 209–210
Popped Amaranth Hemp Seed Salad, 249
Popped Amaranth Rooibos Pizza, 239–240
puddings, 125–126

recovery drinks, 127–129
Recovery Pudding, 126
Rooibos Almond Milk, 268–269

salad dressings, 251–257
salads, 246–251
sauces, 261–267
Sesame Miso Soup, 245
smoothie additions, 217–221
smoothies, 217–226
soups, 244–246
Spicy Black-Eyed Pea Quinoa Pizza, 235–236
Spicy Chocolate Energy Bars, 229–230
Spicy Cocoa Pancakes, 214–215
Spicy Sun-Dried Tomato Marinara Sauce, 266–267
sport drinks, 122–123
sport gels, 123–125
spreads, 261–267
Sunflower Seed Beet Pizza, 237
Sunflower Seed Pâté, 266
Sweet Green Smoothie, 226
Sweet Pepper Hemp Pesto, 267
Sweet Potato Sesame Pizza, 238

Thrive Diet basics, 209–211
Toasted Apple Cinnamon Cereal, 216–217
Tomato Basil Dressing, 256
Tropical Pineapple Mango Smoothie, 223–224

Vegetable Crackers, 259
vegetables, 240–244

Walnut Hemp Burger, 233
Wild Rice Split Pea Pizza, 240
Wild Rice Yam Pancakes, 212

Zucchini Chip Almond Salad, 250
Zucchini Chips, 260
Zucchini Pasta, 243–244

subject index

An "*f*" following a page number indicates a figure on that page.

absorption, 38
açaí, 149–150
acid-forming foods, 52–53, 54–55
acidic environment, 47, 52
acidosis, 47–48, 121
active yeast, 69
adapting
  to change, 85–87
  to Thrive Diet, 87–88
additives, 158–160
adrenal glands, 9–10, 14
advanced glycation end products (AGEs), 46–47
agave nectar, 158
alkaline-forming foods, 48–54, 56–57
alkalizing foods, 121
allergic reaction, 65
almonds, 145–146
amaranth, 39, 139–140
amino acids, 16, 59, 136–137, 151
ancient grains, 67, 285
anemia, 137–138
anti-aging attributes of exercise, 101
antioxidants, 285
anxiety, 20
appetite, 61–62
apple cider vinegar, 159
assimilation, 38
athlete-specific recalibration, 117–118

balsamic vinegar, 159
bananas, 293
berry seed oils, 207
big meals, 17
bioavailability, 45
biological age, 285
biological debt, 70–74, 285
biotin, 276
blender drinks, 78
blood cells, 17
bone health, 55–56
brown rice, 147–148
buckwheat, 39, 140–141

caffeine, 79, 153, 157
calcium, 55–56, 138, 278
calorie, 37
carbohydrate, 57–58, 281–282
cardiovascular exercise, 103
carob, 206
celiac disease, 285
cell reconstruction, 46
cellular regeneration, 23–24, 59
changes, 82–83, 85–87
children, 75–76
chlorella, 150–152, 220, 294
chlorophyll, 48–49, 54, 86–87, 90, 130–131, 150, 152
chocolate flavor, 206
chromium, 278
coconut, 153
coconut oil, 144
coconut water, 293
coffee, 71
cognitive ability, and nutrition, 16–17
cold-pressed oils, 291, 292–293
commercial sport nutrition products, 107
complementary stress, 27–29, 100
complex carbohydrates, 58
conventional farming, 26–27
cooking. See recipes
copper, 278
corn, 66–67
cortisol, 10, 11
cramping, 108–109
cravings, 17–20, 87, 101, 108

dairy, 67–68
dark leafy greens, 130–131
darkness, 81–82
dates, 142–143
deep relaxation, 81–82
detoxification, 151
detoxification symptoms, 87
dietary fat, 59–60
digestion
  acid-forming foods, 54–55
  and energy, 35–36
  nutrient-deficient foods, 37
  nutrient-dense foods, 38
digestive enzymes, 134
dinosaur kale, 131
drinking water, 27
dulse, 63, 132, 208

economics, 98–99
electrolytes, 286
empty food, 286
energy
  cost-free energy, 71–72
  for digesting food, 35–36
  food production requirements, 92–95
  retained energy resources, 39
  shift of energy, 94
  and starchy, high-carbohydrate foods, 37–38
energy bars, 72–73, 90, 120
energy cycle, 93
enjoyment
  of diet, 80
  of exercise, 103–104
  of life, 56
the environment
  and economics, 98–99
  energy requirements of food production, 92–95
  protein production, 95–96
  soil quality, 96–97
  and the Thrive Diet, 97–98
environmental stress, 45
enzyme enhancement, 44–46
essential amino acids, 136–137
essential fatty acids, 16, 43, 134, 221, 283
ethanol, 92–93
exercise
  alkalizing foods, 121
  and anti-aging, 101
  benefits of, 101–102
  cardiovascular exercise, 103
  and complementary stress, 27–28
  fuel sources during exercise, 110*f*
  getting started, 102–105
  level-one activity, 109, 111–112
  level-three activity, 110–111, 113–114
  level-two activity, 109–110, 112–113
  nutrition before exercise, 108–114
  nutrition during exercise, 114–118
  nutrition immediately after exercise, 118–121
  and omega-3, 135
  and personality, 103–104
  and poor nutrition, 100–101
  pre-exercise snack, 109–114
  and proper nutrition, 106–107
  resistance training, 103
  speeding recovery, 106–107
  training and nutrition journal, 104–105
extra-virgin olive oil, 144

farming subsidies, 96
fat accumulation, 13–14
fatigue, 73
fats
  see also oils
  cravings, 17–18
  dietary fat, 59–60
  essential fatty acids, 134, 283
  fatty acids, 43, 59–60, 286
  generally, 282–283
  high-quality fats, 43
  metabolism of, 134–135

trans fats, 289
fatty acids, 43, 59–60, 286
fiber
insoluble fiber, 135
and overeating, 63
soluble fiber, 135
fiber-rich carbohydrates, 41
fibrous vegetables, 131, 161
filberts, 147
flash pasteurization, 53–54
flaxseed, 134–136, 157
flaxseed oil, 145
flour, 163, 205–206
fluids, 78–79
folate (folic acid), 277
folic acid, 277
food allergies, 65
food elimination, 65, 66
food production, 26–27, 92–95
food sensitivities
active yeast, 69
common food sensitivities, 64–65
corn, 66–67
dairy, 67–68
defined, 65
food elimination, 65, 66
gluten, 67
peanuts, 69–70
soy, 68
symptoms, 64
wheat, 67
free radicals, 286
frequent eating, 89
fructose, 16, 287
fruit, 43, 142–143, 162

G Living Network, 296
gas production, 133, 134
getting started
exercise, 102–105
Thrive Diet, 89–90
ginger, 159
glossary, 285–289
glucose, 16, 287
gluten, 67
grains, 147–149, 163
grazing, 165–166
green tea, 153, 295
green tea seed oil, 153–154
greens, 59
grocery shopping, 165
ground water seepage, 27
growth hormone, 101–102
Guayaki, 292

hazelnuts, 147
health as goal, 33
healthy food, importance of, 84–85
hemp, 136–137, 292
hemp oil, 145, 206
hemp protein, 54, 95–96, 136–137
herbs, 163, 201–202
high achiever's syndrome, 29
high-fructose corn syrup, 67
high net-gain nutrition, 34–37, 39–40
high-quality fats, 43
high-temperature cooking, 46–47
hormonal imbalance, 11–12
hydration, 78–79

immune system, 15–16, 152
inflammation reduction, 46–47, 134, 136
insoluble fiber, 135
insoluble fibrous plant matter, 45
iodine, 279
iron, 152, 279

journal, 104–105
juice, 207
junk food, 85

kale, dinosaur, 31
kelp, 132
kid-friendly recipes, 75–76

lactic acid, 121
leafy greens, 130–131
legumes, 42, 133–134, 162
level-one activity, 109, 111–112

level-three activity, 110–111, 113–114
level-two activity, 109–110, 112–113
lifestyle tips
  avoid too many changes, 82–83
  darkness, 81–82
  enjoyment of health pursuit, 80
  healthy food, importance of, 84–85
  mind-body connection, 83–84
  natural light exposure, 80–81
lignans, 287
liquid meals, 120
low-grade metabolic acidosis, 47–48
low-temperature cooked foods, 44–47

maca, 154–156, 219–220, 294
macadamia nuts, 146
magnesium, 279
Maine Coast, 292
malnutrition, 12
manganese, 279–280
Manitoba Harvest, 292
matcha green tea, 153
MCTs (medium-chain triglycerides), 144
meal plans
  generally, 167–168
  using, 89
  week 1, 169–171
  week 2, 172–174
  week 3, 174–176
  week 4, 176–179
  week 5, 179–181
  week 6, 181–184
  week 7, 184–186
  week 8, 186–189
  week 9, 189–191
  week 10, 191–194
  week 11, 194–196
  week 12, 197–199
meditation, 82
melatonin, 82
milk, 67–68
millet, 148
mind-body connection, 83–84
minerals, 63–64, 96–97, 278–281
molybdenum, 280
money, 98
motivation, 25–26
muscle cramping, 108–109
music, 74

natural light exposure, 80–81
naturopathic medicine, 65
net gain, 287
net-gain nutrition, 34–37, 38, 39–40
next-level foods, 149–158
nori, 132
NOW, 293
nutrient-deficient foods, 37
nutrient-dense foods, 38, 60–62, 287
nutrient density, 38
nutrition
  adapting to new way of eating, 86
  and blood cells, 17
  and cellular regeneration, 23–24
  and cognitive ability, 16–17
  and exercise, 106–107
  before exercise, 108–114
  during exercise, 114–118
  immediately after exercise, 118–121
  net-gain nutrition, 34–37, 38, 39–40
  one-step nutrition, 57–60
  pre-exercise snack, 109–114
  primary-source nutrition, 97–98
  training and nutrition journal, 104–105
Nutrition MD, 296
nutritional stress
  defined, 23
  food production, 26–27
  meaning of, 6
  overconsumption of refined food, 24–25
nutritional yeast, 69, 159–160
nuts, 145–147, 163, 202–203

obesity rates, 61
oil dependence, 94

oils, 143–145, 163, 206–207, 292–293
see also fats
olive oil, extra-virgin, 144
omega–3, 134–135, 157, 283
omega–6, 134, 283
O.N.E., 293
one-step nutrition, 57–60, 287
organic farmers, 97
Organics Unlimited, 293
overreaction, of stress-response mechanism, 10

peanut butter, 37–38
peanuts, 69–70
pesticides, 26–27
pH, 47
pH balance, 47–57
phosphorus, 280
photosynthesis, 48
phytonutrient, 287
pituitary gland, 101
placebo effect, 83–84
planning ahead, 165
plant foods
advantages of, 45
bioavailability, 45
enzyme enhancement, 45
plantains, 293
pollutants, 45
positive attitude, 56
positive change, 28–29
post-workout drinks, 107
potassium, 135, 280–281
pre-exercise snack, 109–114
primary-source foods, 97–98, 288
probiotics, 220–221, 288
processed food, 24–25
production stress, 29–30, 31, 117
protein, 53–54, 59, 108, 283–284
protein isolates, 53
protein production, 95–96
pseudograins, 39, 42, 139–141, 162
the psyche, 25
pumpkin seed oil, 145
pumpkin seeds, 137–138
purple sticky rice, 147

quinoa, 39, 141

raw foods, 44–47
recalibration, 77, 88, 117–118, 288
recipes
see also Recipe Index
herbs, 201–202
philosophy, 200–201
soaking nuts and seeds, 202–203
sprouting seeds, 203–205
variations, 205–208
recovery, 2, 81–82, 106–107
recovery test, 3–5
reducing stimuli, 88
refined food, 24–25, 71
resistance training, 103
resources, 290–295
restaurant eating, 166
rice, brown, 147–148
rooibos, 156, 292–293

salads, 90
Salba, 293–294
salt, 62–63, 207–208
Sambazon, 294
sea salt, 207–208
sea vegetables, 132, 162, 292
seaweed, 132
seeds, 42, 134–139, 162, 202–205, 205–206
selenium, 281
sensory system, calibration, 76–77
Sequel Naturals, 294
serotonin, 18–19, 155
sesame seeds, 138–139
shopping list, 161–164
simple carbohydrate, 43, 58, 288
sleep, 12, 81–82
smoothies, 90, 120
snacks
afternoon, on Thrive Diet, 90
best time to consume, 120, 121
pre-exercise snack, 109–114

soaking nuts and seeds, 202–203
soil quality, 96–97
soluble fiber, 135
soy, 68
spelt, 148
spices, 164
sport drinks, 114–116
sport gels, 116–117
sprouted foods, 60, 134
sprouting seeds, 203–205
Stahlbush Island Farms, 295
staple foods (Thrive Diet)
  additives, 158–160
  fruit, 142–143
  grains, 147–149
  legumes, 133–134
  next-level foods, 149–158
  nuts, 145–147
  oils, 143–145
  pseudograins, 139–141
  seeds, 134–139
  vegetables, 130–132
starches, 43–44
starchy vegetables, 132, 161
sterols, 155, 288
stevia, 160, 292–293
stimulation, 30–32, 73, 74, 76
stress
  adrenal glands, 9–10, 14
  change as stress, 85–87
  complementary stress, 27–29, 100
  control and use of, 9
  cortisol, 10, 11
  and depressed moods, 18
  and diet, 73
  environmental stress, 45
  and enzyme destruction, 45
  and fat accumulation, 13–14
  fatigue, 73
  and health problems, 11–12
  and hormonal imbalance, 11–12
  and maca, 155
  nutritional stress. See nutritional stress
  personal account of, 12–15
  and positive change, 28–29
  production stress, 29–30, 31, 117
  psychological stress, 22–23
  and sleep, 12
  spiral, 72*f*, 73–74
  stimulation, 30–32, 73, 74, 76
  symptoms, 16
  and Thrive Diet, 5
  toll of stress, 15–16
  types of stress. See stressors
  uncomplementary stress, 20–27, 100
  and weakened immune systems, 15–16
stress-response mechanism, 10
stressors
  breakdown of stressors, 21*f*
  complementary stress, 27–29, 100
  production stress, 29–30, 31
  uncomplementary stress, 20–27, 100
sunflower seeds, 139
sunlight, 80–81
supplements, 63–64
sweet tooth, 18–19
sweeteners, 163
symptom-treating programs, 33–34

teff, 149
television watching, 75
Thai black rice, 147
Thrive Diet
  adapting to, 87–88
  alkaline-forming foods, 47–57
  appliances needed, 164
  applying the Thrive Diet, 85–88
  biological debt, elimination of, 70–74
  biological resources, fewer required, 26
  and children, 75–76
  and cortisol levels, 74
  and the environment, 97–98
  enzyme enhancement, 44–46
  expected results, 34
  food sensitivities, 64–70
  general guidelines, 89

getting started, 89–90
high net-gain nutrition, 34–37, 39–40
hydration, 78–79
inflammation reduction, 46–47
lifestyle tips, 80–85
and long-term success, 34
low-temperature cooked foods, 44–47
meal plans. See meal plans
nutrient-dense whole foods, 60–62
and nutritional stress, 6
objectives of, 6
one-step nutrition, 57–60
pH balance, 47–57
pH effect, selected foods, 49–51
primary-source nutrition, 97–98
pyramid, 40–44, 58
raw foods, 44–47
recalibration diet, 77, 88
resources, 290–295
shopping list, 161–164
specific guidelines, 89–90
staple foods. See staple foods (Thrive Diet)
starting slowly, 87–88
and stress, 5
traveling and, 164–166
whole foods, 62–64
Thrive Diet pyramid, 40*f*, 40–44, 58
Touch Organic, 295
toxins, 46–47, 54, 86–87
trace minerals, 288–289
see also minerals
training and nutrition journal, 104–105
trans fats, 289
traveling, 164–166
typical North American diet, 51–52

uncomplementary stress
common sources of, 21
described, 20–22
and exercise, 100
motivation, 25–26
nutritional stress, 23–26
and the psyche, 25
psychological stress, 22–23

variations, 205–208
Vega products, 291
vegetables, 41–42, 130–132
vinegars, 163
vitamin A, 273–274
vitamin B1, 274
vitamin B2, 274
vitamin B3, 274–275
vitamin B5, 275
vitamin B6, 275
vitamin B12, 275–276
vitamin C, 276
vitamin D, 80, 276
vitamin E, 277
vitamin K, 277
vitamins, 63–64, 273–277
Vita-Mix, 295

walnuts, 146
water, 79
wheat, 67
white bread, 36–37
white chia, 156–157, 293–294
white tea, 295
whole foods
benefits of, 62–63
defined, 289
and energy needs, 39
nutrient-dense foods, 60–62
nutritional stress-reduction properties, 14
whole grains, 58
wild rice, 141

yeast, 69, 159–160
yerba maté, 117–118, 157–158, 292

zinc, 281